THE KETO LIFESTYLE

Simple 7 Day Meal Plans To Kickstart Your Ketogenic Diet

By

Mary Parrett

Table of Contents

Introduction

More often than not, engaging and persevering in laborious performances to keep you fit and trim would seem to become exasperating. In the end, you will only come to realize that everything you do never makes any sense. Rather than achieving your weight-loss goals, you eventually lose all your patience!

Besides, the several varieties of weight-loss programs dominating in the fitness world today, yet, passing as fleeting fads, only confuse you even more. Additionally, when you cope up strictly with their program guidelines, they only entail great difficulties.

As a resolve, the **THE KETO LIFESTYLE** presents incisively the ketogenic or keto diet as your ultimate solution. Foremost, the meal plans demonstrated herein will be your invaluable strategies on how to control your caloric intakes, promote enhanced fat-burning and metabolic processes in your body, boost the growths of lean muscle mass, or shed off your excessive and unwanted kilos while staying fit in the quickest, safest, and healthiest way possible.

Lest you think warily that this book has a catch, the meal plans and the diet itself will even tolerate you to consume more fats! Yes, you have just read it right—you eat FAT to keep you FIT!

While this may sound like science fiction, you must better believe it. The fat-ness for fitness eating plan is not a myth, and it will never be! It is actually part of the natural metabolic calisthenics of the body. In other words, it is the healthiest alternative that your body necessitates. See for yourself after digesting further the meat of the matter!

Essentially, the unorthodox ketogenic regimen is exclusively a low-carbohydrate and high-fat diet. Vegetable and animal oils, butter, and heavy cream are the usual components in your keto meal plans to provide you with the necessary fats. Therefore, such fats will be the reason for letting you shy away from taking sweets (sugar or glucose-based carbohydrates).

By simply replacing basic carbohydrates with healthy fats, the regimen eventually transforms your body into a virtual fat-burning machine! Hence, since your body will be burning fewer carbohydrates, your cognitive processes heighten because your brain uses up more stored fats for energy; and in no time than you will expect, your appetite decreases, which results in dramatic losses in body weight!

While the keto dietary program restricts strictly carbohydrate-rich foods, it can still allow you to accept generous levels of tolerances. Nonetheless, you ought to measure your meals accordingly in terms of the diet's ideal daily macronutrient intakes or calorie consumptions.

Apparently, you may be forming doubts and misgivings about the regimen by all its specific food restrictions and tolerances. Yet, on the contrary, the old perception that fats are harmful to your health is now fast becoming a yarn. This no longer imposes any precautions with the diet.

Therefore, you can really rule out any thoughts of food deprivation. Besides, you can still feast on your favorite foods while enrolled in the program since you will have several alternatives for their essential ingredients that are as delectable, yet, healthier.

Medical research and science have been helping us to improve our basic understandings of proper nutrition. At this point, we must have already learned that many types of fats can truly be healthy for the body! For all we know, fats definitely manifest major improvements in various health risk factors such as cholesterol and blood sugar levels. Fact is that the keto dietary plan continuously provides a myriad of time-tested health and wellness benefits.

For this reason, several new variations and tweaked adaptations of the keto diet mushroomed but merely flourished as short-lived trends. Generally, they capitalized more on the marketing ploy of weight reduction but compromised the significance of staying fit and healthy.

The Atkins diet, which is also a low-carbohydrate and high fat (LCHF) diet, has been one of the most notable versions of these modifications. However, the only distinctive difference is that the ketogenic diet regulates moderate protein consumptions. In short, it actually focuses to control each macronutrient intake. At any rate, you can then consider the ketogenic diet as an instituted dietary discipline that is more holistic with its working principles and basic concept.

Hereupon these pages contain your fundamental guide towards a deeper understanding of the keto diet. They primarily direct you to learn the principle of attaining the natural and ideal metabolic state of the body through optimal ketosis. Moreover, the book aims to distinguish the keto regimen as an established medical nutrition therapy for eating more fats in order to lose weight. All the information you gained from this book will prepare you towards the proper performances and implementations of the diet.

First, you will know how to calculate for your recommended calorie intake values. These values will be significant in shaping to create your food recipes and meal plans, and eventually, help you stay on course with the diet.

Second, you will have a definite grocery guide of recommended and restricted food groups to help you stick to the regimen. This also enables you to form prudent decisions on choosing your ideal keto meal.

Third, the book provides you with 80 inspiring, delicious, budget-friendly, and easy-to-prepare keto recipes categorized under breakfast, lunch, dinner, snack, and dessert meals. Each recipe will comprise the 7-day meal plan samples across 1,500-, 1,750-, and 2,000- calorie consumptions. Hence, the book covers the range of your healthy weight goals and wellness agenda depending on your recommended or calculated daily calorie consumption.

Exciting as it could ever be, you will most likely have your moments of glory for whipping up your personal recipes or formulating other food preparation variations as soon as you get the hang of practicing the ketogenic diet! You only have to trust and live by the process!

Chapter 1-Knowing Deeper the Ketogenic Diet

Originally, the popular indulgence of the keto diet was for patients afflicted with epilepsy and seizures. However, no one could really determine precisely the working mechanisms of the diet in alleviating or treating seizures. Despite all the formulated theories on how the diet works, the definite assurance for its neurological therapeutic values is the occurrence of metabolic changes that greatly influence the brain's chemical composition.

During the recent past, the keto diet has regained new interests due to its slew of therapeutic potentials. The medical field affirms its feasibility for treating patients diagnosed with diabetes and cancer, as well as people suffering from neurodegenerative diseases, like Alzheimer's disease, Parkinson's disease, and brain damage during a stroke.

In 1921, Dr. Russell Wilder of the Mayo Clinic in Minnesota developed the ketogenic diet, which focuses on a very low consumption of carbohydrates and a high intake of fats. The ketogenic diet derived its terminology from *ketogenesis*, which is the metabolic process of generating sufficient quantities of ketone bodies. This process is a natural alternative function of our body's metabolism that allows us to survive without food intakes for a definite period.

With this specific eating habit, the diet produces a similar effect on fasting, whereby, the body ultimately creates ketone bodies in the liver. During fasting, the level of glucose in the blood decreases (hypoglycemia). Glucose is the major nutrient of muscles, especially the brain. The body would then adapt itself to the deprivation of food, as well as the reduction of glucose by tapping its reserves of energy. Typically, the body draws in the stored fatty tissues, which the liver transforms into ketone bodies.

On average, your body can store hundreds of thousands of calories, which comprise of fats. Thus, your liver produces large quantities of ketone bodies during fasting. After three days into the fast, the energy at the level of neuron cells in the nervous system will be a third of ketone bodies. This denotes that your body will seemingly have an unlimited supply of energy. It now only depends on how long you sustain living through without food. Unfortunately, therefore, a complete fasting plan leads to muscle loss; and obviously, it could not be a feasible and lasting healthy solution.

Under the ketogenic diet, the ketone bodies—sourced from the metabolism or breaking down of fat intakes—enable all your body cells (including neurons) to be functionally flexible. With higher fat and lower carbohydrate consumption, your body incurs lower glucose levels over time. The erstwhile glucose-reliant cells of your body switch automatically to burning ketone bodies for fuel.

Ketone bodies possess uniquely desirable characteristics. In comparison to glucose, burning ketones result in lesser oxidative damages to your cells. In fact, the brain and heart function better with energy sourced from ketone bodies rather than glucose. As such, this also implies that ketones are more effective in generating greater energy than the body does from burning glucose. Hence, ketones are much efficient, safer, and healthier body fuels for your cells to use.

Program Principles & Core Concept

Ketogenesis normally occurs to all of us, particularly when we fast, skip a meal, or simply, lower our carbohydrate or glucose intakes. The minimum lifetime carbohydrate limit seems to be zero, especially if we consume adequate amounts of proteins and fats.[1] It is, therefore, a completely natural state that has allowed humanity to thrive through millennia.

This indicates that ketogenesis suppresses our appetite without experiencing the gnawing pangs of hunger or fasting. Therefore, engaging with a diet rich in fats, yet, less in carbohydrates promotes ketogenesis.

Your principal purpose now in indulging with the ketogenic diet is how to govern your body cells into mobilizing its natural alternative function of shifting into the metabolic process of ketogenesis. This simply means that you should attain a state of optimal ketosis— switching your body's main metabolic function from the processing of carbohydrates to the breaking down of fats to produce ketone bodies for fuel.

In terms of reducing weight, the reduction of carbohydrate intakes is a given and well established. The ketogenic diet is no exception. Not only will the diet allow you to lose weight easily but also, it helps to alter or reverse effectively health risk factors often linked to chronic heart disease (CHD) and diabetes such as *glycemia* (concentrated presence of glucose along the bloodstream), blood *triglycerides* (bad cholesterol in the blood), and various symptoms of inflammatory diseases [2, 0, 0, 0, 0].

Attaining Optimal Ketosis = A-OK!

Switching your body quickly into an optimal state of ketosis heavily depends on your food consumption! High-fat diets are effective for the simple reason that they force your body to trigger undergoing a state of ketosis.

Ketosis is actually a metabolic state wherein your body has an extremely high fat-burning rate. During this state, ketone bodies in your blood begin to increase exponentially. Obviously, your body has no carbohydrates to burn primarily except fats!

Oftentimes, many adherents to the strict ketogenic regimen become very cautious and conscious that their ketone levels in the blood might fall beyond the ideal values. This should not surprise you. **The key to the proper performance of the diet is to avoid all foods derived from starchy sources, or plainly, carbohydrates! You should be restrictive on your carbohydrate intakes and only allow consuming less than 30g daily!**

The standard ketogenic diet actually prescribes at least 5% of calories each day from carbohydrates. We may have different body compositions, so it could be possible that you may achieve your most efficient ketone levels by taking 20g of carbs daily while another individual may consume 40g to reach their optimal state of ketosis.

Nevertheless, 30 grams of carbohydrates per day is the rule of thumb in the keto world. You may wonder how or what a 30-gram of carbohydrate intake looks like. (The 80-recipes for breakfast, lunch, dinner, snacks, and desserts, as well as the different meal plans in this guidebook, will show you how and what).

You may even be afraid of eating leafy greens since you will be dodging carbohydrates like Neo dodging a spray of bullets in the Matrix. Thus, therein lays **the main predicate and purpose of this guidebook—to develop your will and intuition for taking only 30 grams of carbohydrates so you will be more comfortable consuming the nourishing whole foods you need while skipping the junk foods you do not.**

Carbohydrates per se are neither good nor bad. They are merely molecules where carbon bonds with water. However, fiber is a carbohydrate type that never influences blood glucose levels. In the first place, fiber is insoluble and goes through the body undigested. It is only essential for a healthy and normal gut function, where the gut bacteria in the large intestine break them down.

Hence, for a clearer picture of a 30-gram carb comprising whole foods with fiber, you just subtract the fiber from the total carbohydrate value. For instance, if a whole food contains 8 grams of carbs with 5 grams of fiber, you would net 3 grams of carbs.

Equally important is to be cautious with your protein consumptions. Ingesting substantial quantities of protein will cause your body to convert the protein excesses into glucose. Besides, heavy protein consumptions tend to increase insulin levels, which control the metabolism of carbohydrates. In effect, this hinders your goal of achieving optimal ketosis.

In resolving this dilemma of reverting into breaking down of carbohydrates, it would be highly advisable to satisfy your gastronomic cravings with more fats. Although this may sound queer, such a peculiar advice will certainly weave wonders for you!

In principle, consuming more fats allows you to feel fuller. It suppresses abruptly your appetite or curbs your intents of taking more food serving portions. As a result, your high fat regimen will ensure lesser protein and carbohydrate ingestions. In the process, it directly addresses your excessive weight issues. Certainly, your insulin levels drop and your body attains optimal ketosis.

To repeat, maximizing your results under a ketogenic dietary program is to attain the metabolic state of optimal ketosis. The trick is not only to restrict your intakes of carbohydrates but also to be fully aware of partaking proteins. The secret, unbelievably, is to have your fill of fats...lots of fats! Your only problem now is to know how much fats, proteins, and carbohydrates you should take to attain optimal ketosis.

Ketogenesis/Ketosis Macronutrient Model: Ideal Implementation of the Correct Caloric Configuration Consumption

There are six main groups of macronutrients: carbohydrates, proteins, fats, vitamins, minerals, and water. The majority of the daily diets nowadays involve consuming calories with about 50% of carbohydrates, 35% of fats, and 15% of proteins.

Oppositely, the ketogenic diet consists almost exclusively of fats and proteins (at a specific dose per kilogram of your ideal body weight). As previously mentioned, your objective is to draw your energy primarily from fats via ketones and secondarily from glucose reserves.

Therefore, as a standard macronutrient model for undergoing ketogenesis/ketosis, your total DAILY caloric configuration consumption should approximately be as follows:

🍽 **70% to 80% of calories from fats**

🍽 **15% to 25% of calories from proteins**

🍽 **5% to 10% of calories from carbohydrates**

These ketogenic macronutrient ratios are very important and you should always be aware of them. By this caloric configuration[7], it apparently translates to considering the following conditions for your body to reach ketosis:

🍽 **Consume enough fats.**

🍽 **Update the proteins in your food recipes and meal plans regularly.**

▌●▌ Minimize your carbohydrate consumption.

These conditions must always complement each other. They should not go as one without the other. If you consume fewer carbohydrates but also lesser fats, you will be feeling tired constantly and depriving your body of energy. Conversely, if you eat more fats and you do not alter your carbohydrate consumption, you will surely fail and gain more weight due to excess calorie intakes!

Due to this seeming caloric imbalance, it would be necessary to supplement the diet with additional sources of vitamins and minerals. Of course, you should maintain drinking the traditional 6 to 8 glasses of water daily.

Each of the rated caloric percentages helps you to derive your recommended daily calorie intake. You will then know what food to eat and how much of each macronutrient category you should consume based on your specific body composition and lifestyle.

Implementing strictly the ketogenic diet may baffle patients, caregivers, or practitioners alike with its seeming difficulties. This is chiefly due to your presumed time devoted to and spent in planning and measuring your keto meals.

Nonetheless, any unplanned meals will imminently lead to breaking the momentum of your regular requirements for a nutritional balance. Thus, for the regimen's optimum efficiency, always try to consume your measured foods! Always plan before you use! Always apply the keto ratios! Always conform to the keto values!

Keystone Labels for Ketone Levels: Knowing the Kismets of Ketosis

While you follow the standard macronutrient consumptions of a keto diet, you might be unable to know whether your body is in a state of ketosis. During the first week of practicing the keto diet, ketosis can cause unpleasant symptoms such as fatigue, headaches, bad breath (fruity smell), thirstiness, and weakness. Once your body becomes adaptive to it, it would be difficult for you to know whether your liver is actually producing ketone bodies to provide your body with the energy it needs.

Alternatively, you are unsure whether your body has an excess of ketone bodies. An overproduction of ketones promotes *ketoacidosis* (high acidity levels in your blood), which leads further to health complications. Thus, it is indeed important to check or measure your ketone levels.

Typically, ketone bodies manifest in your urine. You can apply the traditional spot test, which uses chemically coated dipsticks you can easily avail from your local pharmacy. If the analyzed urine contains *acetoacetic acid* (ketones), the reactive surface of the dipstick changes its color. The color chart printed on the package has labeled parameters, which allow you to compare the color and determine the approximate amount or concentration of ketone bodies in your urine.

However, dipsticks are generally unreliable since they do not render accurate measurements. They rather leave you clueless about the exact concentration levels and presence of ketones.

More innovative but pricey blood glucose measuring gadgets are more reliable to give you accurate measurements. While most of these devices require pricking your forefinger with a needle for a blood sample, you can readily determine the precise levels of your ketones within seconds.

The following will be your guidelines in interpreting the differently ranged values of ketone concentrations, measured in *mmol/L* (millimoles per liter):

➜ **Below 0.50-mmol/L** denotes a ketone count that is way beyond optimum levels of burning fat. Under this range, your body is not in a state of ketosis but only depicts to have normal levels of ketone bodies.

➜ **Within 0.50 to 1.50-mmol/L** signifies a moderate ketone count, which results in a better metabolism of fats and weight reduction with no deficiencies of insulin. However, this range does not indicate optimum conditions of ketosis. Instead, this only connotes that your body is undergoing a lighter or normal nutritional ketosis.

➜ **Within 1.50 to 3.0-mmol/L** portrays the recommended ketone levels for optimum weight loss. This specific range essentially exhibits the ideal values for attaining a state of optimum nutritional ketosis. Nonetheless, you should be on the lookout when reaching on the verge of a higher ketone level. In all likelihood, you will be at risk of incurring diabetic ketoacidosis. Consult immediately with your doc for further advice.

➜ **Above 3.0-mmol/L** demonstrates achieving neither worse nor better conditions as compared to ketone levels within the 1.5o to 3.0 mmol/L range. Thus, the ketone counts within this range are often negligible values. However, higher ketone levels only imply that your body is either having lesser food intakes or having a serious metabolic issue. For the latter, prompt medical care is necessary.

Just the same, it is never advisable to exceed 80 mg/dL (8-mmol/L) or a dark purple color on the dipstick. If this occurs to you, ask yourself if you have been drinking enough fluids; or better, increase your carbohydrate intake. If you clearly exceed this level, it may be a sign that your body has difficulties with the metabolism of ketones. This situation is very rare, but it requires an immediate examination by your doctor.

The ideal time to measure your ketones is during the beginning of the evening (because during the day, the amount of ketones in your urine is usually low). If you do it during the day, ensure having an empty stomach, or preferably, before breakfast.

Alternatively, choose a time when you are performing your usual daily tasks. Yet, never perform the test right after an intensive activity since your body cells will have a greater need for energy sourced from ketone bodies in your blood.

Actually, attaining the ideal metabolic state of optimum nutritional ketosis is achieving your healthy weight loss goals and wellness agenda. More importantly, it is reaping a host of the regimen's rewards.

Chapter 2-Reaping the Regimen's Remarkable Rewards

Despite the fact that the intended establishment of the ketogenic dietary program was initially for the treatment of seizures, epilepsy, and other issues of the nervous system, legions of individuals have now accepted to practice the regimen with a variety of reasons or goals. Foremost of these goals is to reap the regimen's remarkable reward for losing extra poundage while at the same time gaining more energy.

More significantly, the continued popular practice of the diet stems from a myriad of wellness benefits. For the record, the prestigious European Journal of Clinical Nutrition[8] compiled the following report in June 2013 about the following general health and wellness issues that the keto diet has been dealing with successfully:

♥ **Reducing Rapidly Weighty Weights**[9] – Cutting down on your carbohydrate intake is among the most effective, yet, simplest ways to reduce weight. Research even shows that people indulging in low-carbohydrate and high-fat diets tend to lose more weight quicker compared to most practitioners of low-fat diets (not to mention that low-fat dieters aggressively limit their calorie intakes)!

Aside from the fact that your body virtually becomes a fat-burning machine, the major reason behind this favorable rapid weight reduction outcome is that the keto diet decreases insulin levels. A low insulin level stimulates the appropriate retention of sodium contents in your body. Meaning, your body normally experiences a diuretic effect, inducing urination to drain the excess body fluids. In effect, your kidney starts to rid out excess sodium, which actually causes fluid retention or a temporary fluid weight gain.

♥ **Curbing Cravings and Abating Appetites**[10] – A regular intake of fats suppresses automatically your sweet tooth cravings, as well as your intents for extra servings. Hence, even if you do not try, you will frequently end up consuming only the ideal keto calorie amounts. With a healthier lifestyle that includes physical exercises, along with a declining level of your appetite, they complement the process of reducing your unwanted bulks and bulges!

♥ Optimizing Optimistic Outlooks – Since the diet prompts you to eat fats, your brain consequently sources its energy from the breaking down of fats. Studies, needless to say, show that fat metabolism results in lesser depression and stress symptoms, uplift overall moods, and more satisfaction and happiness in life.

♥ Modifying Symptoms of the Metabolic Syndrome[11] – Over the long term, ketosis helps to reduce the number of health risks and issues by altering or reversing the dreaded *metabolic syndrome*—an aggregation of the following dangerous symptoms:

- Low Levels of High-Density Lipoprotein (HDL)

- High Levels of Low-Density Lipoprotein (LDL)

- High Levels of Triglycerides (TG)

- High Blood Pressure Levels

- High Blood Sugar and Insulin Levels

- Obesity or Destructive Abdominal Fats Buildup

♥ Qualifying Qualitative LDL & Quantitative HDL – The main function of lipoproteins in your body is to convey fatty cholesterols in your bloodstreams. Your *'bad cholesterol'* or LDL transports fats from your liver to the different cells and organs of your body. Your *'good cholesterol'* or HDL carries fats from your body to your liver, which may excrete or reuse them as ketone bodies. For a diet rich in fats, your LDL levels decrease while your HDL levels increase.

In other words, high quantities of HDL enhance fat metabolism while degraded qualities of LDL restrict the circulation of bad cholesterols in your body. Being such the case, this gives rise to balanced cholesterol levels that will prevent incurring risks of various heart ailments and stroke.

♥ Trimming and Taming Triglycerides (TG) – A common indicator of acquiring CHD is incurring high TG-to-HDL ratios. In most cases, your blood triglyceride levels have tendencies of shooting up, especially when you indulge with a low-fat regimen.

Since the keto diet can increase your HDL levels through rich intakes of fats, it only follows that your TG-to-HDL ratios logically decrease. This also means that there will be a constant reduction of fat molecules in your bloodstream.

♥ **Hampering the Happenstance of Hypertension** – High blood pressure, also termed as *hypertension,* is a principal risk factor for many health issues such as CHD, stroke or decreased levels of oxygen in the brain, kidney failure, dementia or other neurodegenerative disorders, and several others. Medical research about the keto diet shows that blood pressure reductions are directly proportionate to reduced consumptions of sugary and starchy carbohydrates.

♥ **Disabling the Development of Diabetes**[11, 12] – A low-carbohydrate intake also results in decreased insulin and blood sugar levels. In short, it prevents the onset of prediabetes conditions, as well as Type-II diabetes mellitus.

Essentially, Type-II diabetes mellitus appears to characterize high blood sugar levels that your body cannot reduce on its own. The reason for your body's difficulty to lower blood sugar levels is commonly due to *insulin resistance*[13], whereby, your body can no longer produce sufficient insulin hormones to keep blood sugar levels down to their normal range.

♥ **Overcoming Obesity**[14] – The recommended macronutrient or caloric consumption values of the regimen result in controlling *insulin spikes* (secretion of insulin) and prevent drastic upswings in your blood sugar levels. Additionally, your regulated calorie intake destroys the accumulation of destructive stored fats in your abdominal cavity. Hence, aside from suppressing of your appetite, the diet prevents you to incur obesity issues while maintaining a healthy weight.

♥ **Curtailing Conceptions of Cancer Cells** –Similar to your body cells, a tumor cell produces energy. It flourishes by usually tapping glucose sourced from starchy carbohydrates to burn at extremely rapid rates compared to other cells in your body. They only weaken and ultimately cease to thrive with an abundance of fats around and a decreased glucose supply.

♥ **Boosting Brainpower & Cognitive Capabilities**[15] – With enhanced blood sugar and balanced cholesterol levels, you will gain optimum blood vessel health. This also indicates that your healthy blood vessels can constantly supply sufficient amounts of oxygen, as well as ketones to your brain cells to burn for energy. Compared to glucose, ketones can prevent your brain cells from undergoing destructive processes of *oxidative stress* (release of free radicals, which results in cellular degeneration), Hence, ketosis reduces your risks of acquiring Alzheimer's disease, Parkinson's disease, and other forms of neurodegenerative dysfunction or mental deterioration.

♥ **Leasing Longer Lives & Leading Lively Lifestyles** – As the keto diet secures a specific macronutrient requirement that provides your ideal daily calorie consumption for general healthcare, it also lowers your chances of developing symptoms of muscle weakness or frailty by about 70%. Thus, you can be as dynamic as you can be. Moreover, since the diet also lessens your risks of developing life-threatening illnesses, you virtually reduce your mortality risks by roughly 20% at any age!

Chapter 3- Starting & Sticking to the Program's Proper Performances

Fundamentally, the ketogenic dietary program is a holistic medical nutrition therapy. It involves crucially particular participants from the various medical disciplines.

Your entire medical team may include a neurologist/physician who has the vast experiences in prescribing the diet; a certified nurse who is knowledgeable enough about the cause and effects of the regimen; and, a professional dietitian who shall coordinate with the regular implementation of the dietary program.

In addition, more assistance and support may need the services of a licensed pharmacist who shall advise about the specific dosages of prescribed carbohydrate values and medicines, and perhaps, a registered medical social practitioner who shall collaborate with your family. Finally, for the safe and proper program performance, other medical caregivers, as well as your immediate family members should have the necessary understanding and information about the various important aspects of the regimen.

As you get to start practicing the keto dietary plan, always heed the wise advice of availing the guidance and close supervision of your medical adviser. Inevitably, there are somehow risks of complicating health matters during your initiation to the program aside from acquiring the keto flu and other side effects.

For instance, if you are suffering from Type-1 diabetes mellitus, you should forego proceeding to attain optimal ketosis since it can pose further harm to your health. Nevertheless, if ketone bodies are indeed present in your bloodstream, ensure that your blood sugar should be at normal levels.

Having a normal blood sugar level indicates that your body can be at normal ketosis, similar to the states of ketosis exhibited by healthy practitioners of a strict low-carbohydrate regimen. On the contrary, having a high blood sugar level with an abundance of ketones only denotes that insulin levels are extremely low.

Although non-diabetics do not typically suffer from these risky blood sugar levels, they may acquire *diabetes acidosis*, or ketoacidosis, which could be life-threatening. When such condition happens, your body requires more insulin injections.

However, prudence will dictate that you should seek medical advice, especially when you are not sure at all. Gaining higher ketone levels for the sake of losing weight will never be worth the risk for individuals with Type-1 diabetes mellitus.

Regimen's Requirements & Regulations

Practicing the keto diet may eventually take several forms. Thus, it is only prudent to repeat some significant details discussed previously to etch in mind and avoid confusion. **However, its standard practice remains to comprise a daily carbohydrate consumption of not more than 30 grams.**

As you keep your carbohydrates restricted, you will be inclined to consume often meals derived principally from fats, dairy, vegetables, and nuts. Specifically, your meals should be a composition of ample amounts of animal and vegetable fats, including proteins sourced from dairy produce, vegetables, and nuts.

More importantly, follow strictly the formulaic daily ketogenic nutritional value proportions of 70%-80% calories from fats, 15%-25% calories from proteins, and 5%-10% calories from carbohydrates! You should also bear in mind that a high-protein intake would prevent your body from reaching optimal nutritional ketosis. Thus, set your daily protein consumptions with respect to the percentage of your body fat and lean body mass. To calculate:

You first figure out the percentage of your body fat.

Your body fat percentage X your weight = your amount of fat.

Your lean body mass = your weight – your amount of fat.

The daily amount of your protein intake = 0.8 X your lean body mass, in pounds

**If you prefer using metric units and calculations, then you multiply
1.8 by your lean body mass in kilograms.**

Rationalizing Rated Ratios

The rated caloric ratios in a keto diet are alternative calculations for your
required daily caloric consumptions. Oftentimes, these rated ratios are
importantly applicable when taking into account the intensities of your
daily activities.

The ketogenic diet uses the most common caloric ratios of 4:1 and 3:1.
In details, a 4:1 ratio denotes a keto diet comprising 4 grams of fats for
every gram of proteins including carbohydrates.

In short, for every 5 grams of consumed food, you will have 4 grams of
fats and a gram of proteins/carbohydrates. Hence, a 4:1 keto diet
consists of 80% fats (that is, 4÷5=80%) and 20% proteins/carbohydrates
(that is, 1÷5=20%). Similarly, a 3:1 keto diet consists of 75% fats (that is,
3÷4=75%) and 25% proteins/carbohydrate (that is, 1÷4=25%).

As you will notice, the ketogenic rated ratios compare the quantities of
fats, proteins, and carbohydrates expressed in grams, which is a weight
measure. This is because you will be measuring your keto foods by their
weight using a gram scale.

If you will compare fats, proteins, and carbohydrates in accordance to
their provided number of calories instead of the provided number of
grams, the concluding ratio would be slightly different. This stems from
the fact that fats provide your body with more calories (9 calories per
gram) compared to protein and carbohydrates (4 calories per gram).

For instance, you require consuming 360 calories. To provide your body
with 360 calories from proteins/carbohydrates, you need to consume 90
grams of proteins/carbohydrates (that is, 360÷4=90). Yet, to receive the
same number of calories from fats, you need to consume only 40 grams
of fats (360÷9=40).

Fats actually provide your body with the same amount of calories with
much lesser weight or mass since it is denser calorically compared to

proteins and carbohydrates. Such being the case, the keto meals tend to appear smaller than those standard meals, despite providing exactly the same number of calories.

If you were on a 4:1 keto diet ratio, then that would mean a 90%-calorie in your diet comes from fat. Think again. Lest you confuse yourself further by wondering how it could be 80% fats and 90% fats at the same time, it is indeed 80% fat if you measure the diet by weight and 90% fat if you measure it by calories.

Put in mind that a 4:1 keto ratio signifies 4 grams of fat for every gram of proteins/carbohydrates. Thus, 4 grams of fat, which gives 9 calories per gram, provides a sum of 36 calories (that is, 4 x 9 = 36); 1 gram of proteins/carbohydrates, which gives 4 calories per gram, provides a sum of 4 calories (that is, 1 x 4 = 4). Alternatively, the calorie ratio of fat to proteins/carbohydrates is 36:4. This implies that each 40-calorie intake, 36 calories come from fat while 4 calories come from proteins/carbohydrates. Hence, 90% of the calories come from fat (that is, 36÷40=90%) while 10% come from proteins/carbohydrates (4÷40=10%).

Chapter 4-Grocery Guide

As you launch your keto dietary program but you are quite unsure where to take off and what foods to consume, the following food-shopping list comprises the most notable and recommended keto diet foods. The list, categorized under the major food groups is, by no means, extensive. Nonetheless, it directs you towards staying on course with your keto program.

Always remember to choose products rich in fats and low in carbohydrates when you are shopping for food items with your ketogenic diet. Fats are your source of energy!

However, always be careful! Read the product labels well. Labels of the different food products would surprise you to see how much sugar and carbs they contain!

In the beginning, you will have to work extra hard to find what you need, but you will get the hang of it over time. Like any other discipline or training, the keto regimen has its shares of difficulties at the start, especially when picking the right item from the grocery shelf. By practicing it with frequency, everything becomes easy as counting 123 and reciting ABC!

It would be a prudent advice though to stick to selecting and consuming mostly fresh and real foods. Real foods denote organic, unprocessed, and natural foods. Although processed or canned goods can be beneficial and convenient in a pinch, particularly when you wish on taking anything quickly with fewer carbohydrate contents, nothing beats consuming much healthier foods that are at their most natural form.

Inclusive Items for Constant Consumption (Recommended & Restricted Rations)

Basic Beverages

[Be cautious with drinks containing sweeteners since they may consist of carbohydrates.]
- **Coffee** *(with unsalted butter or cream, but no milk)*
- **Carbonated or sparkling water**
- **Distilled water**

Dairy Doses

[Preferably, opt for full fat, raw & organic dairy products. If you like to reduce weight, it is wise to skip all dairy items except for unsalted butter for your coffee.]
- **All low-carb cheeses** *(i.e., asiago, blue, brie, burrata, cheddar, Colby, cottage, cream, feta, Fontina, goat, gorgonzola, Gouda, Gruyere, Havarti, Manchego, Monterey Jack, mozzarella, Muenster, parmesan, pepper jack, provolone, ricotta, Romano, Roquefort, and Swiss)*
- **Butter**
- **Clarified butter/ghee**
- **Cream**
- **Greek yogurt**

Elemental Eggs

[Ideally, choose raw, organic, and free-ranged produces.]
- **Chicken**
- **Duck**
- **Goose**
- **Pheasant**
- **Quail**
- **Turkey**

Healthy Herbs & Spice Selections

[Herbs and spices, especially pre-made spices, are critical since they all contain many carbohydrates. Hence, note carefully their values in nutrition labels.]

Fresh Fruits

[Fruits are optional and are dependent on weight and health. While some cannot tolerate fructose, others remain slim and fit with it. Stick to typically low-fructose fresh fruits.]
- **Avocado**
- **Berries**
- **Carambola/Starfruit**
- **Cherry**
- **Coconut**
- **Grapefruit**
- **Lemon/Lime**
- **Casaba melon**
- **Prickly pear**
- **Olives (black/green)**

Favored Flours

[Since the ketogenic diet restricts all types of grains, only consider gluten-free or all other nut flours.]
- **Almond**
- **Coconut**
- **Hazelnut**
- **Macadamia**
- **Pecan**
- **Walnut**

Meaty Meals

[Enjoy liberally the fat and skin of grass-fed and organic meats.]
- **Bacon** *(if possible, charcuterie bacon with the least sugar and without nitrites/nitrates)*
- **Biltong/jerky meat** *(strips of sun-dried cured meat)*
- **Cold cuts & delicatessen meats**
- **Cured meats** *(with the least sugar content & without unknown curing agents and chemicals)*
- **Game** *(domestic/wild)*
- **Livestock** *(veal, pork, mutton, hogget & beef)*
- **Offal** *(internal parts)*
- **Pemmican** *(dried meat cuts mixed with melted fat)*
- **Poultry**
- **Sausages** *(with only meat & spices and without fillers/extenders like sugar, soya, rusk, rolled oats & gluten)*

Notable Nuts

[Avoid European chestnuts since they are steep with net carbs.]
- **Almond**
- **Brazil**
- **Cashew**
- **Coconut**
- **Hazelnut**
- **Macadamia**
- **Peanut**
- **Pecan**
- **Pine**

Veggie Viands

[Limit your choices to low-carb vegetables]
- **Artichoke**
- **Asparagus**
- **Aubergine** *(brinjal, eggplant, garden egg & mad apple)*
- **Bell peppers**
- **Broccoli**
- **Bok choy**
- **Cabbage**
- **Carrot**
- **Cauliflower**
- **Celery**
- **Cucumber**
- **Garlic**
- **Green beans**
- **Kale**
- **Lettuce** *(Batavian, Butterhead, buttercrunch, Chinese, cos or Romaine & loose-leaf)*
- **Mushrooms**
- **Onions**
- **Pepper** *(green)*
- **Radish**
- **Shallots**
- **Snow/sugar snap peas**
- **Spinach**
- **Brussels sprouts**
- **Squash** *(summer, spaghetti & vegetable marrow)*
- **Swiss chard**
- **Tomato**
- **Zucchini**

- **Pistachio**
- **Sacha Inchi/Inca nut**
- **Walnut**

Optimum Oils & Fundamental Fats
- **Animal lard & fats**
- **Avocado oil**
- **Beef tallow**
- **Butter**
- **Coco cream/milk/oil**
- **Crème fraîche & other creams** *(heavy, whipped & sour)*
- **Macadamia oil**
- **Mayonnaise** *(must be homemade, using the proper oils)*
- **Nut butter**
- **Olive oil**
- **Schmaltz/duck fat**

Pantry Picks
- **Bouillon cubes/broth stocks** *(i.e., vegetable, beef, pork, fish & chicken)*
- **Canned/bottled low-carb vegetables** *(i.e., beans, greens, pickles & sauerkraut, etc. with no added sugars)*
- **Canned processed meats** *(i.e., corned beef, luncheon meat, Vienna sausage, etc.)*
- **Canned seafood** *(i.e., anchovies, crab, salmon, sardines, shrimp & tuna)*
- **Canned tomatoes** *(juice, paste, sauce, dried or whole fruit)*
- **Extracts** *(vanilla, lemon, almond, etc., but avoid those with sugar)*
- **Sauces & seasonings** *(gluten-free and with no added sugars or thickeners)*
- **Xanthan gum** *(for binding & thickening)*

Seed Sources
- **Chia**
- **Flaxseed/linseed**
- **Hemp**
- **Pumpkin**
- **Sesame**
- **Sunflower**

Suited Sweeteners

[Use only sweeteners with low glycemic index (GI), which measures the amount of blood sugar raised by food. Use sparingly inulin, sucralose, tagatose, and xylitol. Skip aspartame, maltitol, monkfruit *(Luo Han Guo)*, saccharine, fructose syrup & high sugar alcohols.]
- **Allulose**
- **Erythritol**
- **Stevia**

Supported Seafood

[The keto diet supports global sustainable fishing practices; thus, as much as possible, fish and seafood should be under the list of Southern Africa Sustainable Seafood Initiative (SASSI).]
- **Abalone**
- **Anchovy**
- **Angelfish** *(Atlantic pomfret)*
- **Calamari** *(Cape Hod squid, baby calamari)*
- **Crab** *(fiddler, pea, oyster & soft-shell)*
- **Dorado** *(dolphinfish or mahi-mahi)*
- **Eel** *(kingklip, New Zealand, pink cusk)*
- **Hake/cod**
- **Herring** *(Atlantic, Baltic, redeye round)*
- **Lobster** *(East Coast rock)*
- **Mackerel** *(Atlantic, king, queen & Spanish)*
- **Mussel** *(black, blue, Chilean blue, Chinese, Mediterranean blue, green-lipped & white)*
- **Oyster** *(Pacific & Cape Rock)*
- **Salmon** *(blackfish, blueback, Cohoe, redfish, salmonid, sockeye,*
- **Sardines**
- **Scallop** *(Peruvian)*
- **Seabream** *(black bream, Hottentot, slinger)*
- **Shrimps/prawns** *(Kiddi, Indian)*
- **Snoek** *(barracuda)*
- **Sprat** *(Brisling sardine)*
- **Squid** *(Patagonian, Argentine shortfin, Cape Hope, European & Humboldt flying)*
- **Stockfish** *(shallow-water Cape Hake)*
- **Trout** *(rainbow)*
- **Tilapia**
- **Tuna** *(Albacore, yellowfin, skipjack)*
- **Yellowtail**

NOTE: *When you consumed all the appropriate ketogenic food items, yet, you do not seem to shed off your excess weight, you must have been consuming too much proteins or dairy foods, nuts, and fruits. Thus, maintain your ideal keto macronutrient consumption.*

Abbreviations

Measurements

c	cup
g	gram
kg	kilogram
l	liter
lb	pound
ml	milliliter
oz	ounce
pt	pint
tsp	teaspoon
tbsp	tablespoon

Special Diet Information

VEG	Vegetarian
V	Vegan
GF	Gluten-Free
DF	Dairy-Free
NF	Nut-Free

Chapter 5-Bountiful Breakfasts

1-Choco Chip Whey Waffles

Diet Specs: GF | VEG | DF

Yield: 4-waffles/2-servings

Serving Portion: 2-waffles

Preparation Time: 10 minutes

Cooking Time: 6 minutes

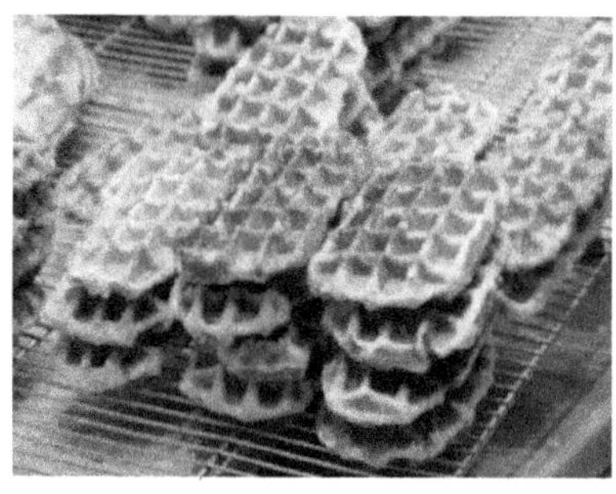

Ingredients:

2-tbsp organic coconut oil

2-tbsp coconut sugar

4-tbsp chocolate whey protein powder

⅓-cup almond flour

A pinch of salt

½-tsp baking powder

½-cup almond milk

2-pcs eggs

Directions:

1. Mix all the ingredients in the blender to obtain a homogenous paste.

2. Preheat your waffle iron. Pour the waffle dough in the iron and cook each waffle for 3 minutes.

Nutritional Values per Serving:

Calories: **423** | Fat: **32.8**g | Protein: **26.5**g | Total Carbohydrates: **8.3**g | Dietary Fiber: **2.9**g | Net Carbohydrates: **5.4**g

2-Coco Cinnamon-Packed Pancakes

Diet Specs: GF| VEG | NF | DF

Yield: 4-pancakes/2-servings

Serving Portion: 2-pancakes

Preparation Time: 30 minutes

Cooking Time: 5 minutes

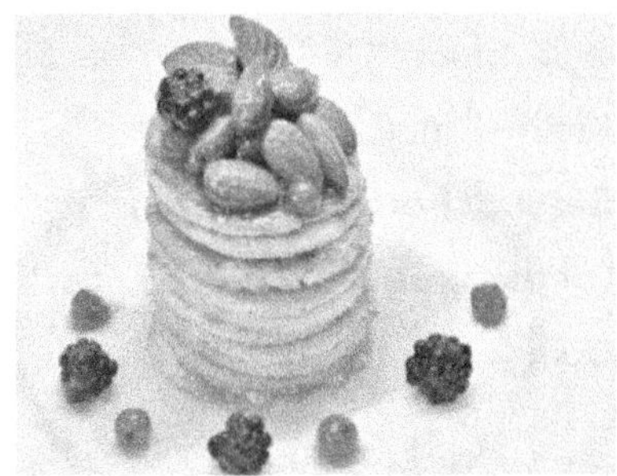

Ingredients:

2-pcs eggs

2½-tbsp organic coconut flour

¼-cup milk substitute with hydrogenated vegetable oil (or almond milk)

1-tbsp baking soda

½-tbsp cinnamon

½-tbsp baobab powder

2-tbsp organic coconut flower syrup

Directions:

1. In a salad bowl, mix the coconut flour, baobab powder, cinnamon, and baking soda.

2. Add the beaten eggs, the almond milk, and the coconut syrup. Let the dough rest for 30 minutes.

3. Cook the pancakes in a hot pan with coconut oil.

4. Dress the pancakes with raspberries/blueberries or almonds.

Nutritional Values per Serving:

Calories: **392** | Fat: **32.5**g | Protein: **20**g | Total Carbohydrates: **11.3**g | Dietary Fiber: **6.4**g | Net Carbohydrates: **4.9**g

3-Magdalena Muffins with Tart Tomatoes

Diet Specs: GF | VEG

Yield: 4-muffins/2-servings

Serving Portion: 2-muffins

Preparation Time: 10 minutes

Cooking Time: 20 minutes

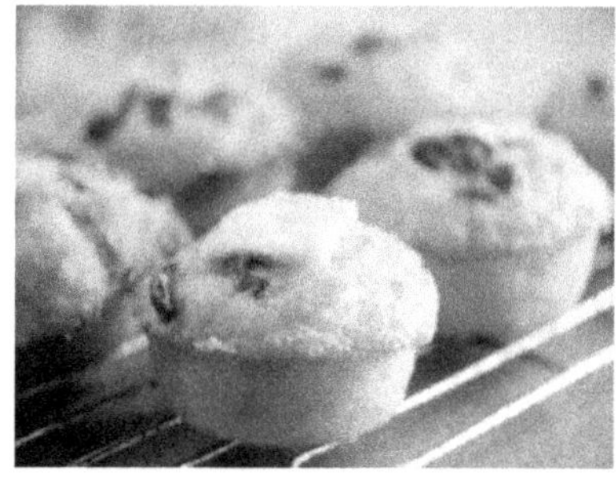

Ingredients:

2½-tbsp whole-wheat flour

2½-tbsp almond flour

1-tbsp yeast or baking soda

A dash of salt, pepper, and paprika

2-pcs eggs

1-tbsp organic cashew nuts

1-tbsp hemp oil

2½-tbsp soymilk

⅓-cup feta cheese, diced

1⅓-cup dried tomatoes, without oil and sliced into small pieces

Directions:

1. Mix the wheat flour, almond flour, yeast, and spices.

2. Then add eggs, cashews, oil, and soymilk.

3. Mix well to obtain a smooth paste. Add the feta and tomatoes.

4. Mix well and pour the dough into muffin pans previously greased with coconut oil.

5. Bake for 20 minutes at 350°F.

Nutritional Values per Serving:

Calories: **405** | Fat: **33.3**g | Protein: **20.3**g | Total Carbohydrates: **11**g | Dietary Fiber: **4.9**g | Net Carbohydrates: **6.1**g

4-Spinach Shoots Mediterranean Medley

Diet Specs: GF | VEG | NF

Yield: 2-servings

Serving Portion: 1 serving bowl

Preparation Time: 10 minutes

Cooking Time: 1 minute

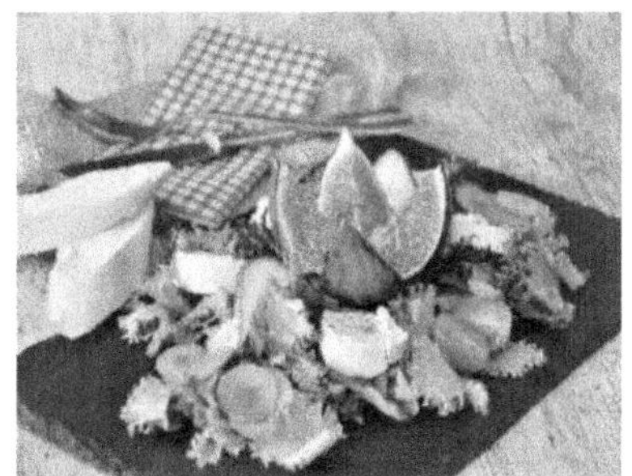

Ingredients:

½-cup spinach shoots

2-tbsp quinoa

¼-cup avocado, sliced

1-tbsp fresh goat cheese

1-tsp agave syrup, gluten-free

¼-cup dried blackberries

1-pc fig

1-tsp pumpkin seeds puree

Directions:

1. Arrange the spinach shoots, cooked quinoa, and avocado on a large plate.

2. Mix the goat cheese, agave syrup, and dried blackberries.

3. Make 4 small cuts in the fig so that you can open it and insert the goat cheese mixture.

4. Spread your fig on the spinach shoots. Sprinkle over with pumpkin seed puree.

Nutritional Values per Serving:

Calories: **308** | Fat: **26**g | Protein: **15.4**g | Total Carbohydrates: **9.7**g | Dietary Fiber: **6.5**g | Net Carbohydrates: **3.2**g

5-Romantic Raspberry Power Pancake

Diet Specs: GF | V | DF

Yield: 2-pancakes/one serving

Serving Portion: 2-pancakes

Preparation Time: 5 minutes

Cooking Time: 10 minutes

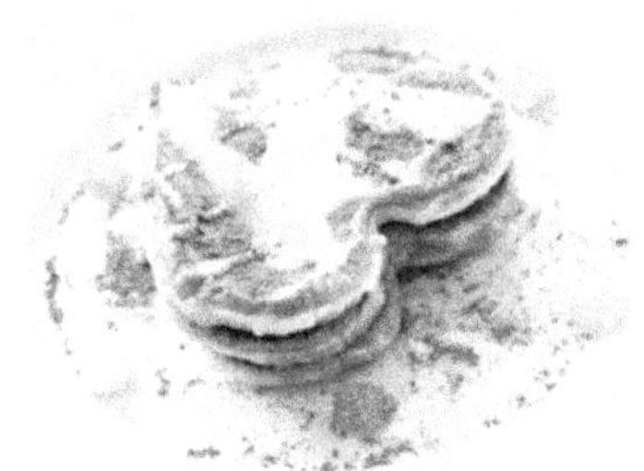

Ingredients:

2-tbsp raspberries, crushed

2-tsp almond flour

1-tbsp yeast or baking soda

1-tbsp vegan protein powder

2-tbsp soymilk

1-tbsp coconut oil

Directions:

1. Mix the crushed raspberries and dry ingredients.

2. Pour the milk and mix well to obtain a homogenous mixture.

3. Cook the pancakes for 2 minutes on each side using a little coconut oil in a pan. Flip the pancake when small bubbles appear.

4. Dress with almonds or nuts.

Nutritional Values per Serving:

Calories: **323** | Fat: **25.3**g | Protein: **15.7**g | Total Carbohydrates: **12**g | Dietary Fiber: **3.8**g | Net Carbohydrates: **4.8**g

6-Spinach Sausage Feta Frittata

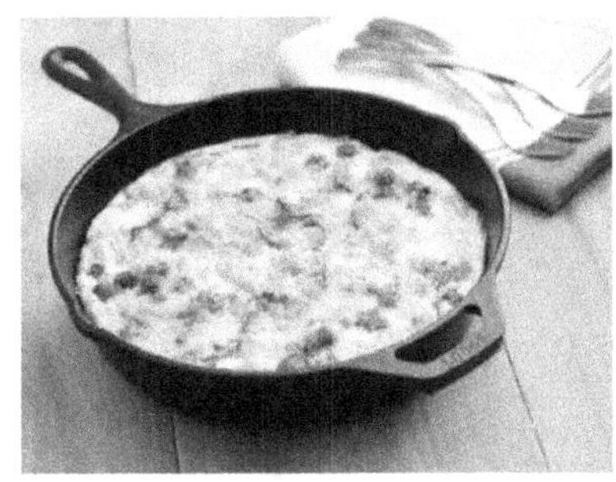

Diet Specs: GF

Yield: 6-frittata wedges/6-servings

Serving Portion: 1-frittata wedge

Preparation Time: 15 minutes

Cooking Time: 30 minutes

Ingredients:

10-oz. spinach, frozen, thawed, drained, and chopped

12-oz. sausage, sliced into small pieces

½-cup feta cheese, crumbled

½-cup almond milk, unsweetened

½-cup heavy cream

¼-tsp. ground nutmeg

½-tsp. salt

¼-tsp. black pepper

12-pcs eggs, whisked

Directions:

1. Place the sausage in a medium-sized mixing bowl. Break the spinach up into the same bowl as the sausage.

2. Sprinkle the cheese over the mixture. Toss lightly until fully combined. Lightly spread the mixture onto a greased 13" × 9" casserole dish, or greased muffin cups.

3. In a larger bowl, blend the almond milk, cream, nutmeg, salt, and pepper with the eggs, and mix well until fully combined.

4. Gently pour the mixture into the dish or muffin cups until for about ¾ full. Bake at 375°F for about 50 minutes (for the casserole), or 30 minutes (for the muffin cups), or until fully set.

Nutritional Values per Serving:

Calories: **295** | Fat: **22.9**g | Protein: **18.5**g | Total Carbohydrates: **4.6**g | Dietary Fiber: **1**g | Net Carbohydrates: **3.6**g

7-Mayonnaise Mixed with Energy Egg

Diet Specs: GF | VEG | NF

Yield: one serving

Serving Portion: 1 serving bowl

Preparation Time: 2 minutes

Cooking Time: 5 minutes

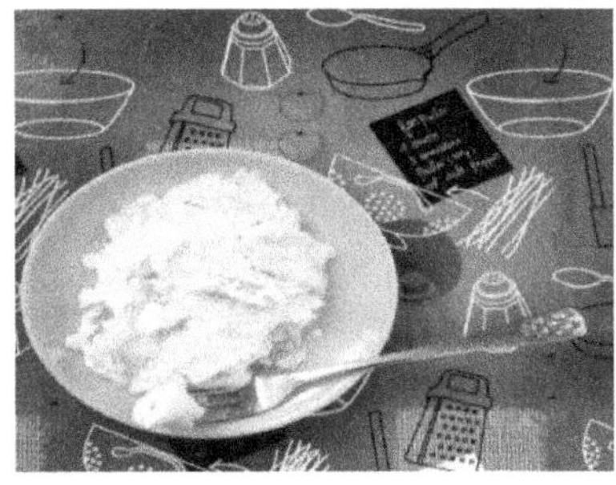

Ingredients:

2-tbsp organic mayonnaise, gluten-free

1-pc large egg

1-tbsp butter

Directions:

1. Mix the mayonnaise and egg in a medium-sized bowl until fully combined.

2. Melt the butter in a non-stick skillet. Pour the egg mixture, and cook until set. Scrape the egg and all remaining fat onto a serving plate. Serve immediately.

Nutritional Values per Serving:

Calories: **295** | Fat: **22.7**g | Protein: **18.8**g | Total Carbohydrates: **3.8**g | Dietary Fiber: **0.1**g | Net Carbohydrates: **3.7**g

8-Avocados atop Toasted Tartiné

Diet Specs: GF | VEG | NF

Yield: 2-tartinés/2-servings

Serving Portion: 1-tartiné

Preparation Time: 10 minutes

Cooking Time: 5 minutes

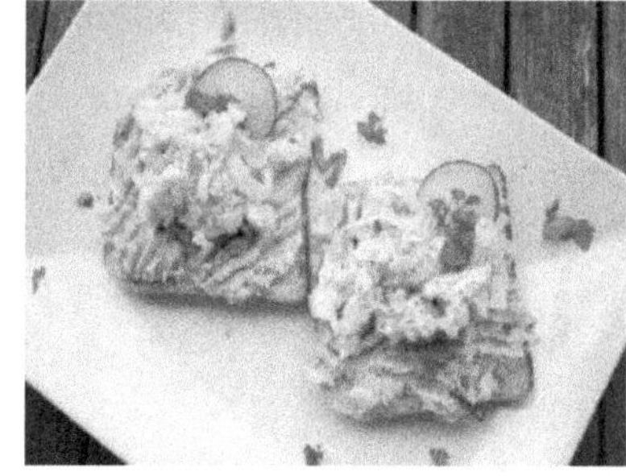

Ingredients:

2-slices bread, gluten-free

½-pc small avocado, thinly sliced

1-tbsp fresh cheese

1-tsp lemon juice

A dash of salt and pepper

1-tsp chia seeds for garnish (optional)

Directions:

1. Toast lightly the bread slices.

2. Carefully arrange the avocado slices on each bread slice. Drizzle with the lemon juice. Spread the fresh cheese. Sprinkle with a dash of salt and pepper. Top with garnish.

TIP: If you like a richer breakfast, you can serve this slice of bread with a slice of hard-boiled egg. You can also garnish the avocado toast with the watercress and chili flakes for a kick of early morning freshness.

Nutritional Values per Serving:

Calories: **268** | Fat: **22.4**g | Protein: **13.5**g | Total Carbohydrates: **8.9**g | Dietary Fiber: **6.7**g | Net Carbohydrates: **3.2**g

9-Fish Fillet & Perky Potato Cheese Combo

Diet Specs: GF | NF | DF

Yield: 2-servings

Serving Portion: 1 serving plate

Preparation Time: 15 minutes

Cooking Time: 10 minutes

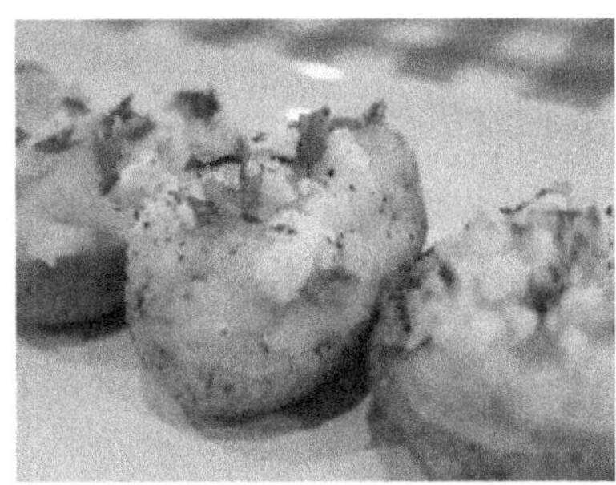

Ingredients:

1-tbsp olive oil

1-pc large potato, cooked and thinly sliced

¼-cup lean white cheese

½-tsp herbs of your choice

3.5-oz. herring fillet, steamed and sliced in half

½-tsp flaxseed oil or coconut oil

A dash of salt and pepper

Directions:

1. Heat a non-stick pan with olive oil. Add the potato slices and cook until browned.

2. Season the white cheese with salt, pepper, and herbs of your choice.

3. Arrange the potatoes equally between two plates. Top with the cheese and herring fillets. Garnish with a drizzle of flaxseed oil.

TIP: Fill in your sautéed potatoes with your favorite ingredients such as fresh onions, parsley or an egg.

Nutritional Values per Serving:

Calories: **298** | Fat: **24.9**g | Protein: **14.2**g | Total Carbohydrates: **6.5**g | Dietary Fiber: **3.2**g | Net Carbohydrates: **4.3**g

10-Cream Cheese Protein Pancake

Diet Specs: GF | VEG | NF

Yield: 4 x 6" diameter pancakes/2-servings

Serving Portion: 2-pancakes

Preparation Time: 10 minutes

Cooking Time: 12 minutes

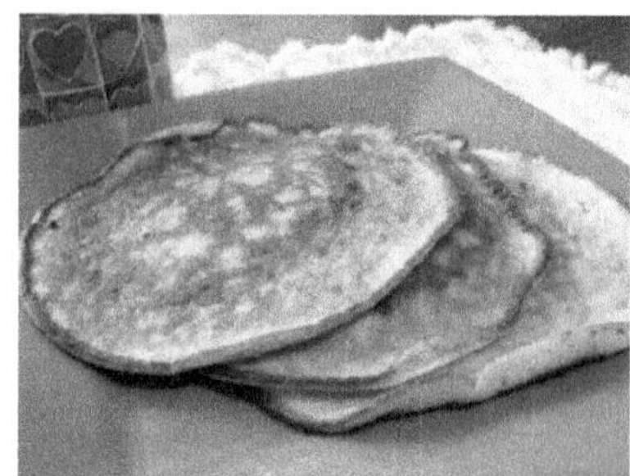

Ingredients:

2-pcs eggs

2-oz cream cheese

1-packet sweetener

½-tsp cinnamon

1-tbsp butter

Directions:

1. Combine all the ingredients except the butter in a blender. Blend until smooth. Let the batter stand for 2 minutes to allow the bubbles to settle.

2. Grease slightly a hot pan with ¼-tbsp butter. Pour ¼-batter into the pan. Cook for about 2 minutes until turning golden. Flip the pancake and cook for 1 minute on its other side.

3. Repeat the same cooking procedure with the remaining batter. Serve with fresh berries of choice and sugar-free syrup.

Nutritional Values per Serving:

Calories: **340** | Fat: **28.1**g | Protein: **16.2**g | Total Carbohydrates: **8.1**g | Dietary Fiber: **3.8**g | Net Carbohydrates: **4.3**g

11-Veggie Variety with Peanut Paste

Diet Specs: GF | VEG | DF

Yield: one serving

Serving Portion: 1 serving bowl

Preparation Time: 15 minutes

Cooking Time: 15 minutes

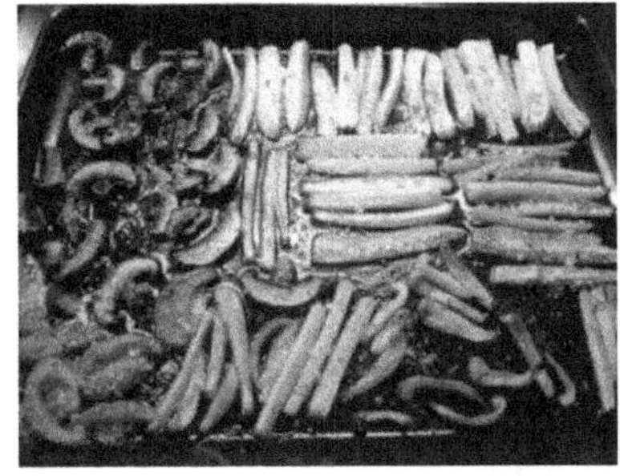

Ingredients:

1-bulb small onion, thinly sliced

¾-cup broccoli, sliced into quarters

1-pc small carrot, sliced into quarters

½-pc green pepper, thinly sliced

5-pcs mushrooms, sliced into quarters

A dash of salt, pepper, and powdered chili

2-tbsp peanut butter, dairy-free

2-tbsp. soy sauce, gluten-free

1-tbsp agave syrup (or honey), gluten-free

¼-cup red cabbage, thinly sliced

Directions:

1. Pour a little water in a heated skillet and cook the onions until they are transparent. Add the broccoli, carrot, pepper, and mushrooms. Cook for 10 minutes until tender. (Add a little water if the pan is too dry). Season the veggies with a dash of salt, pepper, and chili.

2. For the sauce, mix the peanut butter with the soy sauce, agave syrup, and 3 tbsp water.

3. To serve, incorporate the red cabbage. Garnish the dish with the sauce.

TIP: To lessen the calories, the dish uses water instead of oil. If you use oil, preferably coconut oil, you increase the calories by 100.

Nutritional Values per Serving:

Calories: **349** | Fat: **28.7**g | Protein: **18.4**g | Total Carbohydrates: **10.8**g | Dietary Fiber: **6.5**g | Net Carbohydrates: **4.3**g

12-Avocado Aliment with Egg Element

Diet Specs: GF | VEG | NF | DF

Yield: 2-servings

Serving Portion: 1-halved stuffed avocado

Preparation Time: 8 minutes

Cooking Time: 20 minutes

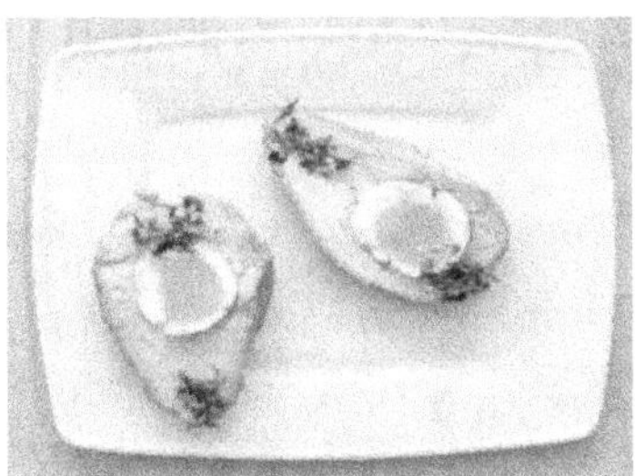

Ingredients:

1-pc egg, whisked

1-pc avocado, halved, pitted, and removed slightly with flesh

A dash of sea salt and pepper

1-tbsp parsley, chopped

1-tsp cayenne pepper

Directions:

1. Preheat your oven to 375°F.

2. Pour the egg gently into each halved avocado. Remove the excess liquid.

3. Place the stuffed avocado in a baking tray. Bake for 20 minutes.

4. Season the preparation with sea salt, parsley, and cayenne pepper.

Nutritional Values per Serving:

Calories: **275** | Fat: **23.8**g | Protein: **11.8**g | Total Carbohydrates: **10.7**g | Dietary Fiber: **4**g | Net Carbohydrates: **3.4**g

13-Pumpkin Pancakes

Diet Specs: GF | VEG | DF

Yield: 6-pancakes/3-servings

Serving Portion: 2-pancakes

Preparation Time: 10 minutes

Cooking Time: 30 minutes

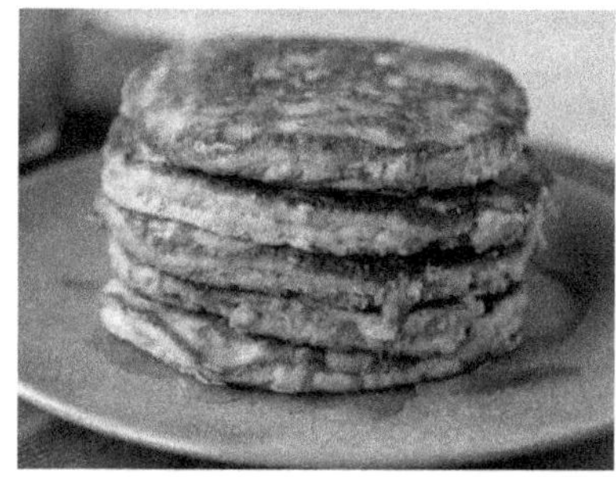

Ingredients:

1-tsp vanilla extract

1-cup coconut cream

3-pcs eggs

2-tbsp egg whites

½-cup pumpkin puree

5-packs sweetener

4-tbsp ground flax seed

4-tbsp ground hazelnuts or hazelnut flour

1-tsp yeast or baking powder

1-tbsp black tea powder

1-tbsp. coconut oil for cooking

Directions:

1. Whisk together the first five liquid ingredients for half a minute until they become frothy. Mix the dry ingredients in a separate bowl.

2. Combine both the dry and liquid ingredients to obtain a batter. (Add water, as necessary if the mixture is too thick.)

3. Grease a saucepan with a teaspoon of coconut oil. Ladle in the first pancake.

4. Cover the pan and cook for 3 minutes. Flip and cook the other side.

5. Repeat the cooking process until using up all the batter.

Nutritional Values per Serving:

Calories: **200** | Fat: **16.4**g | Protein: **11**g | Total Carbohydrates: **5.2**g | Dietary Fiber: **3**g | Net Carbohydrates: **2.2**g

14-Whole-Wheat Plain Pancakes

Diet Specs: VEG | NF | DF

Yield: 2-pancakes/1-serving

Serving Portion: 2-pancakes

Preparation Time: 5 minutes

Cooking Time: 12 minutes

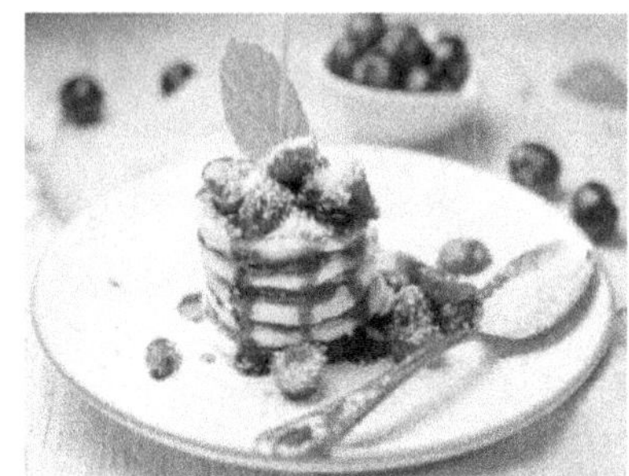

Ingredients:

2-pcs eggs

4-tbsp whole-wheat flour

½-tsp yeast or baking soda

⅓-cup sunflower oil

1-tbsp coconut oil for cooking

Directions:

1. Mix all the ingredients in a bowl until obtaining a smooth consistency.

2. Pour the coconut oil in a pan placed over medium heat. Cook for 3 minutes until browned. Flip and cook the other side.

3. Serve hot and garnish with fresh fruits of your choice such as blueberries, strawberries or raspberries, nuts, and coconut flakes.

TIP: You can mix some blueberries in the batter to create delicious blueberries pancakes.

Nutritional Values per Serving:

Calories: **329** | Fat: **27.6**g | Protein: **16.1**g | Total Carbohydrates: **5.4**g | Dietary Fiber: **1.3**g | Net Carbohydrates: **4.4**g

15-Blueberries Breakfast Bowl

Diet Specs: GF | V | NF | DF

Yield: one serving

Serving Portion: 1 serving bowl

Preparation Time: 35 minutes

Cooking Time: 0 minutes

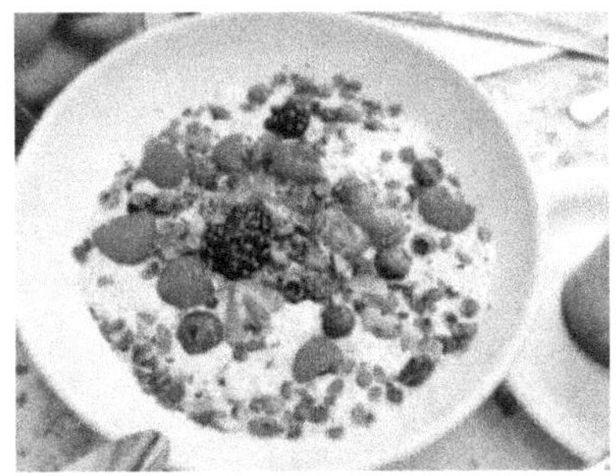

Ingredients:

1-tsp chia seeds

1-cup almond milk

¼-cup fresh blueberries or fresh fruits

1-pack sweetener for taste

Directions:

1. Mix the chia seeds with the almond milk. Stir periodically.

2. Place in the fridge to cool for 30 minutes, and then serve with fresh fruit. Enjoy!

TIP: For an even better taste, let it sit in the fridge for a night and add fresh fruits in the morning.

Nutritional Values per Serving:

Calories: **202** | Fat: **16.8**g | Protein: **10.2**g | Total Carbohydrates: **9.8**g | Dietary Fiber: **5.8**g | Net Carbohydrates: **2.6**g

16-Feta-Filled Tomato-Topped Oldie Omelet

Diet Specs: GF | VEG | NF

Yield: one serving

Serving Portion: 1 omelet

Preparation Time: 5 minutes

Cooking Time: 6 minutes

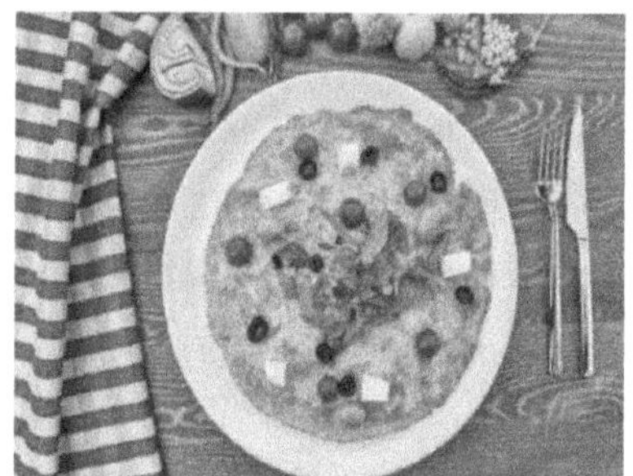

Ingredients:

1-tbsp coconut oil

2-pcs eggs

1½-tbsp milk

A dash of salt and pepper

¼-cup tomatoes, sliced into cubes

2-tbsp feta cheese, crumbled

Directions:

1. Beat the eggs with the milk, salt, pepper, and the remaining spices.

2. Pour the mixture into a heated pan with coconut oil.

3. Stir in the tomatoes and cheese. Cook for 6 minutes or until the cheese melts.

TIP: Add your favorite spices to the omelet for more fun.

Nutritional Values per Serving:

Calories: **335** | Fat: **28.4**g | Protein: **16.2**g | Total Carbohydrates: **4.5**g | Dietary Fiber: **0.8**g | Net Carbohydrates: **3.7**g

17-Ave Avocado Super Smoothie

Diet Specs: GF | VEG

Yield: one serving

Serving Portion: 1 serving bowl

Preparation Time: 10 minutes

Cooking Time: 1 minute

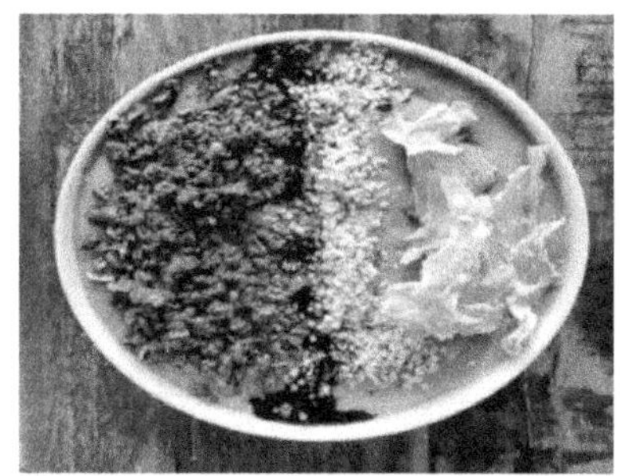

Ingredients:

½-cup Greek yogurt

7-oz. frozen avocados

½-cup water

½-tsp vanilla powder

1-tsp each chia seeds, chocolate chips, and peanut butter for garnish

Directions:

1. Mix all the ingredients. You can also crush them in the blender.

2. Pour the smoothie into a bowl and garnish to your taste with fruits, seeds or nuts.

Nutritional Values per Serving:

Calories: **398** | Fat: **33.1**g | Protein: **20**g | Total Carbohydrates: **15.5**g | Dietary Fiber: **10.6**g | Net Carbohydrates: **4.9**g

18-Hearty Hodgepodge

Diet Specs: GF | NF | DF

Yield: one serving

Serving Portion: 1 serving bowl

Preparation Time: 5 minutes

Cooking Time: 25 minute

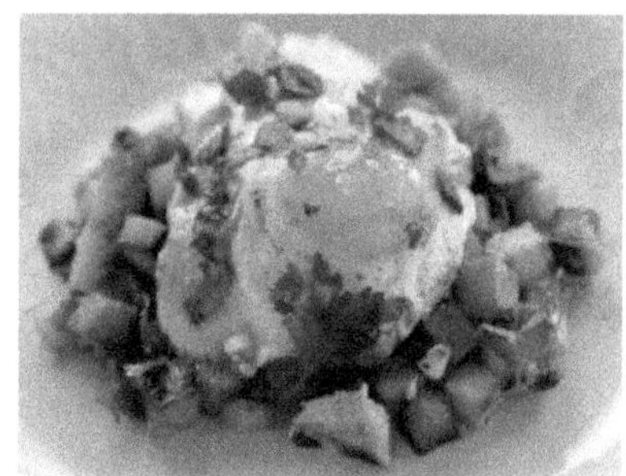

Ingredients:

1-bulb small onion, diced

1-tbsp coconut oil

1-tbsp bacon bits

1-pc medium zucchini, diced into squares

1-tbsp parsley or chives, chopped

¼-tsp. of salt

1-pc large egg, fried

Directions:

1. Sauté the onion with coconut oil in a pan placed over medium heat. Add the bacon, stirring frequently until both onion and bacon turn slightly brown.

2. Add the zucchini, and cook for 15 minutes. Remove from heat and transfer the preparation in a serving bowl. Sprinkle over the parsley.

3. To serve, top the dish with the fried egg.

Nutritional Values per Serving:

Calories: **290** | Fat: **24**g | Protein: **14.6**g | Total Carbohydrates: **6.7**g | Dietary Fiber: **3.1**g | Net Carbohydrates: **3.6**g

19-Chocolate Chia Plain Pudding

Diet Specs: GF | VEG | NF

Yield: 3-servings

Serving Portion: 1 serving bowl

Preparation Time: 55 minutes

Cooking Time: 0 minutes

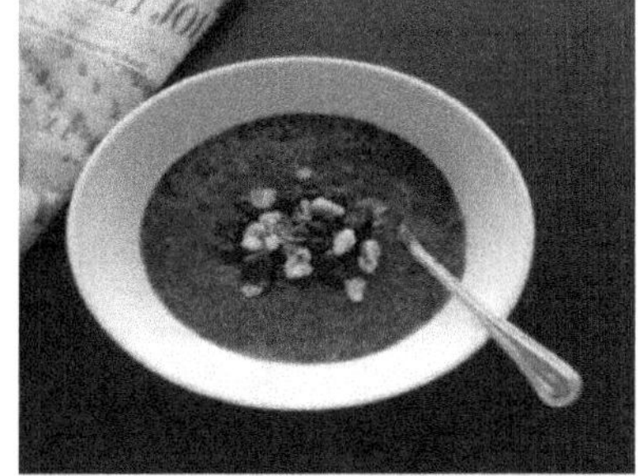

Ingredients:

3-tbsp chia seeds

2-cups water

¼-cup whey chocolate protein

½-cup Greek yogurt, sugar-free

¼-cup linseeds, roasted

1-tbsp cocoa powder, unsweetened

1-packet sweetener (optional)

Directions:

1. Mix the chia seeds with water and let stand for 20 minutes. Stir occasionally.

2. Once the chia seeds are well inflated, add all the other ingredients and mix again.

3. Place in the fridge for 30 minutes before serving.

TIP: Serve with raspberries or blueberries. For a vegan variant, it is possible to use a vegetable yogurt and chocolate vegetable protein.

Nutritional Values per Serving:

Calories: **370** | Fat: **28.7**g | Protein: **22.3**g | Total Carbohydrates: **10.8**g | Dietary Fiber: **5.2**g | Net Carbohydrates: **5.6**g

20-Seasoned Sardines with Sunny Side

Diet Specs: GF | NF | DF

Yield: one serving

Serving Portion: 1 serving bowl

Preparation Time: 5 minutes

Cooking Time: 10 minutes

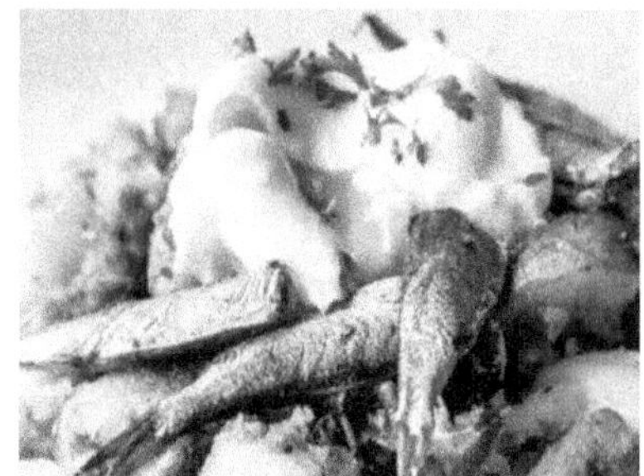

Ingredients:

2-oz. sardines in olive oil

2-pcs eggs

½-cup arugula

¼-cup artichoke hearts, diced

A pinch of salt

A dash of black pepper

Directions:

1. Preheat your oven to 375°F.

2. Place the sardines in an oven-ready stoneware bowl. Add the eggs on top of the sardines. Top the eggs with the arugula and artichokes. Sprinkle with salt and pepper.

3. Bake for 10 minutes until the eggs cook through.

Nutritional Values per Serving:

Calories: **255** | Fat: **21**g | Protein: **13.5**g | Total Carbohydrates: **4.9**g | Dietary Fiber: **1.8**g | Net Carbohydrates: **3.1**g

Chapter 6-Luscious Lunch

1-Pulled Pepper-Lemon Loins

Diet Specs: GF | NF | DF

Yield: 4-servings

Serving Portion: 1 chicken loin

Preparation Time: 15 minutes

Cooking Time: 360 minutes

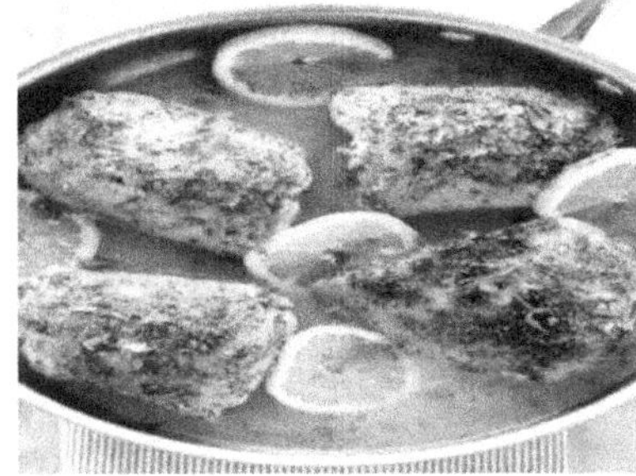

Ingredients

½-stick of butter

1-pc large lemon, sliced

1-pc green pepper, chopped

1-tbsp garlic, minced

2-tbsp olive oil

1-tbsp salt

1-tsp dried thyme

½-tbsp Dijon mustard

3-lbs. (4-pcs) chicken tenderloins

1-cheddar cheese slice, shredded

4-leaves romaine lettuce

Directions:

1. Combine the butter, lemon, pepper, garlic, oil, salt, thyme, and mustard in your slow cooker. Switch the slow cooker on high and melt the butter.

2. Add the chicken; ensure to coat the chicken with the butter mixture.

3. Cook on low for 6 hours or on high for 4 hours. Add the cheese and let it sit for 15 minutes on low.

4. To serve, place the chicken over a bed of lettuce leaves.

Calories: 280 | Fat: 23.3g | Protein: 14g | Total Carbs: 4.1g | Dietary Fiber: 0.6g | Net Carbs: 3.5g

Nutritional Values per Serving:

Calories: **280** | Fat: **23.3**g | Protein: **14**g | Total Carbohydrates: **4.1**g | Dietary Fiber: **0.6**g | Net Carbohydrates: **3.5**g

2-Shrimps & Spinach Spaghetti

Diet Specs: GF | NF | DF

Yield: 2-servings

Serving Portion: 1 serving plate

Preparation Time: 5 minutes

Cooking Time: 8 minutes

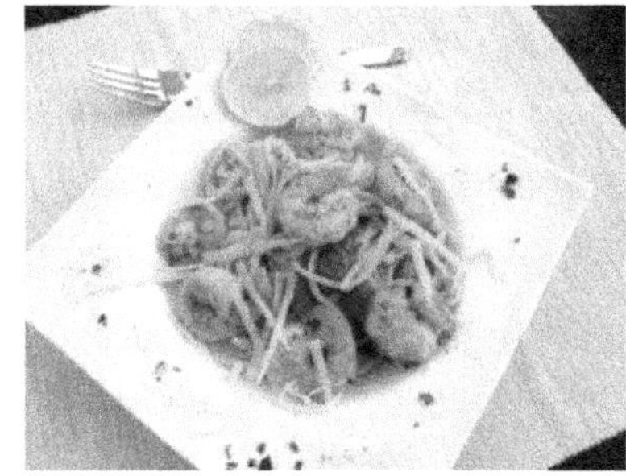

Ingredients:

8-tbsp vegetable broth

1-cup low carb spaghetti, rinsed and drained

1-pc leek, cut into strips

1⅓-cup frozen peas

1⅓-cup fresh spinach leaves

¼-lb. shrimp, pre-cooked

1-tbsp lemon zest

1-pc green pepper, finely chopped (divided, per serving)

2-pcs basil leaves (divided, per serving)

1-pc lemon (divided, per serving)

Directions:

1. Pour the vegetable broth in a wok and cook for 5 minutes. Add the leeks, peas, spinach, and shrimp. Cook further for 5 minutes.

2. Add the spaghetti, and continue cooking for 2 minutes. Remove quickly from heat and pour into a bowl, mix with lemon zest.

3. Divide the pasta equally between two plates. To serve, garnish with the pepper, basil leaves, and lemon.

Nutritional Values per Serving:

Calories: **425** | Fat: **33**g | Protein: **25**g | Total Carbohydrates: **15.7**g | Dietary Fiber: **10.4**g | Net Carbohydrates: **5.3**g

3-Single Skillet Seafood-Filled Frittata

Diet Specs: GF | NF | DF

Yield: 4-frittata wedges/4-servings

Serving Portion: 1 frittata wedge

Preparation Time: 2 minutes

Cooking Time: 18 minutes

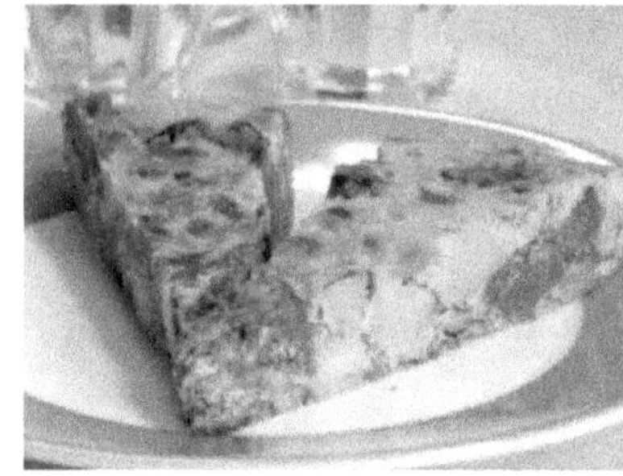

Ingredients:

1-pc green pepper

¼-pc lime, squeezed for juice

1-tbsp coconut flour

1-tbsp sesame oil

1-tbsp soy sauce, gluten-free

1-tbsp coconut oil

3-bulbs fresh onions, chopped

½-clove garlic, minced

¼-cup prawns, raw

1⅓-cup mussels, deshelled

2-pcs eggs, whisked

Directions:

1. Preheat your oven to 475°F. Meanwhile, make the sauce by combining the first five ingredients in a mixing bowl. Mix thoroughly until fully combined. Set aside.

2. Melt the coconut oil in a small skillet and fry the onions. Add the garlic, prawns, and mussels. Cook for 10 minutes until the prawns turn pink.

3. Stir in the eggs. Place the skillet in the oven and bake for 5 minutes.

4. Slice the frittata in four slices and serve with the sauce.

Nutritional Values per Serving:

Calories: **459** | Fat: **38.2**g | Protein: **22.9**g | Total Carbohydrates: **8.7**g | Dietary Fiber: **3**g | Net Carbohydrates: **5.7**g

4-Poultry Pâté & Creamy Crackers

Diet Specs: GF | NF

Yield: one serving

Serving Portion: 3-crackers topped with pate

Preparation Time: 15 minutes

Cooking Time: 35 minutes

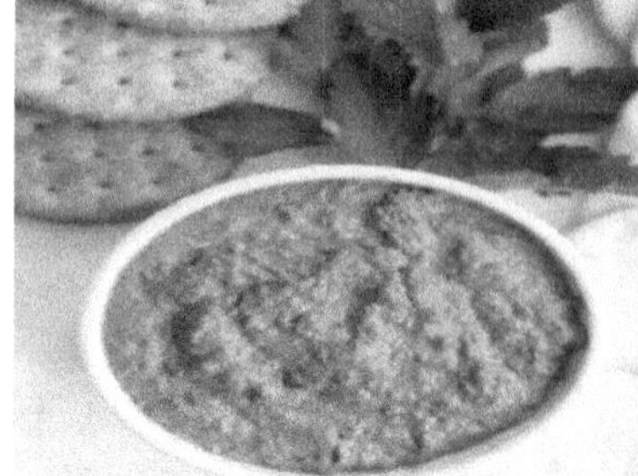

Ingredients:

3.5-oz. chicken livers

3-tbsp butter, softened

1-tsp. Italian seasoning

A pinch of salt and pepper

3-pcs unsalted creamy crackers, gluten-free

Directions:

1. Place all the ingredients in a blender except the crackers. Blend to a smooth paste consistency.

2. Serve with the crackers.

TIP: Instead of crackers, you can use radish slices.

Nutritional Values per Serving:

Calories: **437** | Fat: **36.4**g | Protein: **21.9**g | Total Carbohydrates: **5.5**g | Dietary Fiber: **0**g | Net Carbohydrates: **5.5**g

5-Chickpeas Carrots Curry

Diet Specs: GF | VEG | NF

Yield: one serving

Serving Portion: 1 serving bowl

Preparation Time: 5 minutes

Cooking Time: 25 minutes

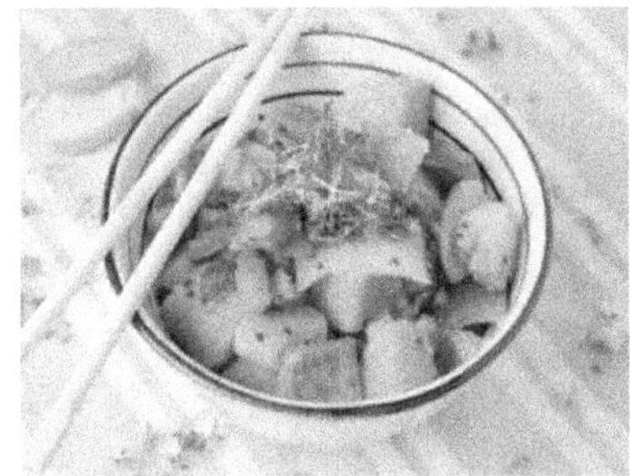

Ingredients:

½-bulb onion, finely chopped

½-pc carrot, sliced into cubes

½-tsp coconut oil

¼-cup chickpeas

½-tsp tomato paste

3-tbsp light soy cream

½-tsp turmeric powder

⅛-bunch fresh coriander

A pinch of salt, pepper, and sweet paprika

Directions:

1. Sauté the onions and carrots for 5 minutes with coconut oil in a skillet.

2. Add the chickpeas, tomato paste, soy cream, turmeric, coriander, and spices. Mix well and cook for 10 minutes.

3. Cook the rice for 10 minutes in boiling water. Serve the konjac rice with the vegetable curry and chickpeas.

Nutritional Values per Serving:

Calories: **380** | Fat: **30.9**g | Protein: **18**g | Total Carbohydrates: **14.4**g | Dietary Fiber: **10.7**g | Net Carbohydrates: **3.7**g

6-Baked Broccoli in Olive Oil

Diet Specs: GF | VEG | NF

Yield: 3-servings

Serving Portion: 1 serving bowl

Preparation Time: 5 minutes

Cooking Time: 25 minutes

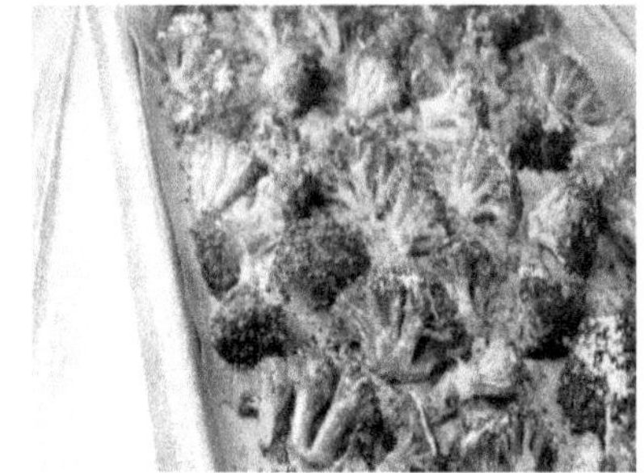

Ingredients:

1½-lbs broccoli florets

¼-cup olive oil

3-tsps garlic, minced

2-tbsp fresh basil, chopped

½-tsp red chili flakes

¾-tsp kosher salt

Zest of ½-pc lemon

Juice of ½-pc lemon

⅓-cup parmesan cheese

Directions:

1. Preheat your oven to 425°F.

2. Arrange the broccoli florets in a baking sheet lined with parchment paper.

3. Season the broccoli with olive oil, chopped fresh basil, minced garlic, kosher salt, red chili flakes, zest and juice of half a lemon each.

4. Sprinkle parmesan cheese over the broccoli. Place the sheet in the oven to bake for about 25 minutes.

Nutritional Values per Serving:

Calories: **484** | Fat: **39.2**g | Protein: **26.7**g | Total Carbohydrates: **21.6**g | Dietary Fiber: **16.8**g | Net Carbohydrates: **4.8**g

7-Bunless Bacon Burger

Diet Specs: GF | NF

Yield: 4-burgers/4-servings

Serving Portion: 1-bacon burger

Preparation Time: 8 minutes

Cooking Time: 37 minutes

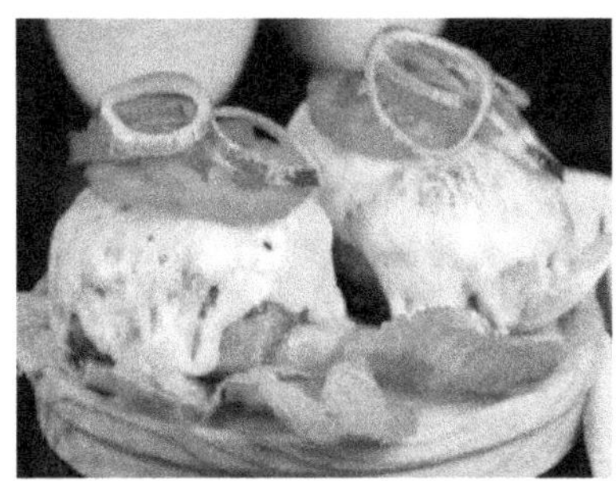

Ingredients:

1½-lbs. ground beef

2-tbsp olive oil

2-tbsp bacon bits

4-oz. pepper jack cheese

1-bulb onion, sliced crosswise

8-leaves romaine lettuce

A dash of salt and pepper

Directions:

1. Form the ground beef into four patties. Cook for 4 minutes with olive oil on a skillet placed over medium heat. Flip the patties to cook the other sides. Set aside.

2. Using the same skillet, stir-fry the bacon bits for 5 minutes until crispy.

3. Use the lettuce leaves as buns. Place each patty on a leaf and top with the bacon bits. Sprinkle a dash of salt and pepper. Top each burger with the cheese to melt.

Nutritional Values per Serving:

Calories: **435** | Fat: **36.3**g | Protein: **21.7**g | Total Carbohydrates: **6.1**g | Dietary Fiber: **0.7**g | Net Carbohydrates: **5.4**g

8-Smoky Sage Sausage

Diet Specs: GF | NF | DF

Yield: 4-patties/4-servings

Serving Portion: 1-patty

Preparation Time: 5 minutes

Cooking Time: 8 minutes

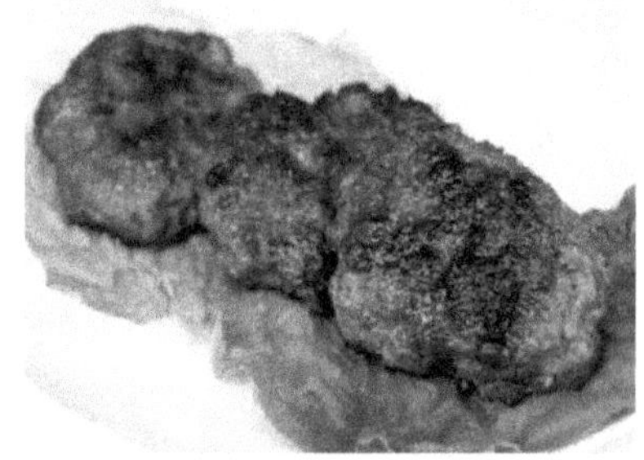

Ingredients:

2-tbsp sage, chopped

2-packets sweetener

1-tsp salt

1-tsp maple extract

1-lb. ground pork

½-tsp black pepper

¼-tsp garlic powder

⅛-tsp cayenne pepper

Directions:

1. Combine all the ingredients in a large mixing bowl.

2. Form patties from the mixture.

3. Put the patties in a skillet placed over medium heat. Cook for 4 minutes until cooked through. Flip the patties to cook on the other side.

Nutritional Values per Serving:

Calories: **170** | Fat: **13.2**g | Protein: **8.4**g | Total Carbohydrates: **5.3**g | Dietary Fiber: **1**g | Net Carbohydrates: **4.3**g

9-Steamed Salmon & Salad Bento Box

Diet Specs: GF | NF

Yield: 2-bento boxes

Serving Portion: 1 bento box

Preparation Time: 10 minutes

Cooking Time: 0 minutes

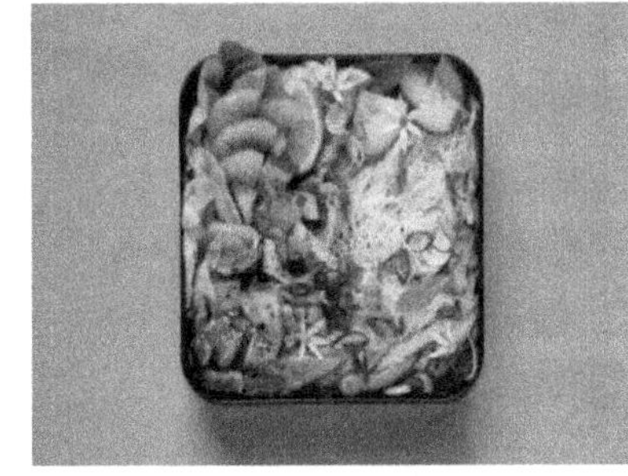

Ingredients:

2-pcs salad heads

1-cup carrot, grated

¼-cup cucumber, sliced

1-pc green pepper, thinly sliced

4-cups marinara pasta, rinsed, drained, and cooked for 2 minutes in boiling water

½-lb. salmon, steamed

2-pcs lemons

2-pcs eggs, boiled and sliced

1-tsp chia seeds

4-tbsp yogurt, sugar-free

1-tsp turmeric powder

½-pc lemon, zest

2-tbsp mint, minced

A pinch of pepper

Directions:

1. Divide equally the first eight ingredients between two bento boxes. Sprinkle the arrangements with chia seeds.

2. Mix the rest of the ingredients to make the sauce. Pack the sauce separately.

TIP: Tofu or minced meat is an option for fish while cucumber noodles are for pasta.

Nutritional Values per Serving:

Calories: **391** | Fat: **30.4**g | Protein: **24.9**g | Total Carbohydrates: **11.8**g | Dietary Fiber: **7.3**g | Net Carbohydrates: **4.5**g

10-Stuffed Spaghetti Squash

Diet Specs: GF | NF

Yield: 2-servings

Serving Portion: 1-halved stuffed squash

Preparation Time: 30 minutes

Cooking Time: 30 minutes

Ingredients:

1-pc spaghetti squash, halved and pitted

1-tsp olive oil

½-cup bacon strips, grilled

3-cups ground beef

1-pc green pepper, thinly sliced

½-bulb onion, sliced into cubes

1-tsp garlic powder

1-tsp paprika

A pinch of salt and pepper

1-cup cheddar cheese, grated

Directions:

1. Rub the squash halves with oil, and bake for 30 minutes at 350°F.

2. Meanwhile, roast the bacon in a saucepan placed over high heat. Stir in the onion and pepper. Add the beef and spices. Season the mixture with salt and pepper, and cook for 15 minutes, stirring regularly. Set aside.

3. Remove the flesh of the cooked squash by scratching with a fork. Mix the flesh with the meat mixture. Add the cheese, and put the mixture in the frayed squash.

4. Return the stuffed squash to the hot oven, and bake for 10 minutes.

TIP: The skin of the squash is thin and hard, so feel free to scrape deep to get the most flesh. You can use avocado instead of squash.

Nutritional Values per Serving:

Calories: **404** | Fat: **33.2**g | Protein: **20.3**g | Total Carbohydrates: **7**g | Dietary Fiber: **1**g | Net Carbohydrates: **6**g

11-Prawn Pasta

Diet Specs: GF | NF | DF

Yield: 3-servings

Serving Portion: 1 serving plate

Preparation Time: 10 minutes

Cooking Time: 12 minutes

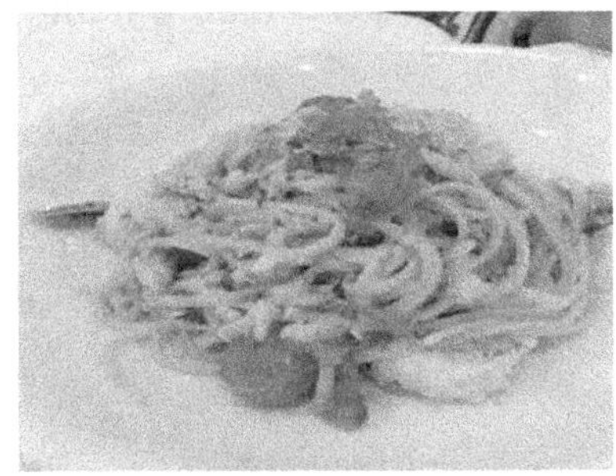

Ingredients:

1-tsp sesame seeds

1-pc lime

½-pc green pepper, thinly sliced

2 tbsp coconut flour

2-tbsp sesame oil

1-tbsp soy sauce, gluten-free

2-heads small cabbages

6-bulbs small onions, chopped

1-cup prawns, steamed

3-cups low-carb pasta, rinsed, drained, and cooked for 2 minutes in boiling water

8-pcs small radishes, sliced into 4-pieces for garnish

½-pc avocado, sliced for garnish

Directions:

1. Combine the first six ingredients in a bowl to make the pasta sauce. Set aside.

2. Cook the cabbage for 10 minutes in a pan with a little water and soy sauce. Add the onions and prawns. Cook for 2 minutes.

3. Arrange the pasta in a plate, topped with the prawn mixture, pasta sauce, and the garnishing.

TIP: You can replace shrimp with feta and sesame seeds with chia seeds.

Nutritional Values per Serving:

Calories: **393** | Fat: **32.8**g | Protein: **19.7**g | Total Carbohydrates: **14.9**g | Dietary Fiber: **10.1**g | Net Carbohydrates: **4.8**g

12- Tasty Tofu Carrots &Cauliflower Cereal

Diet Specs: GF | VEG | NF | DF

Yield: one serving

Serving Portion: 1 serving bowl

Preparation Time: 20 minutes

Cooking Time: 20 minutes

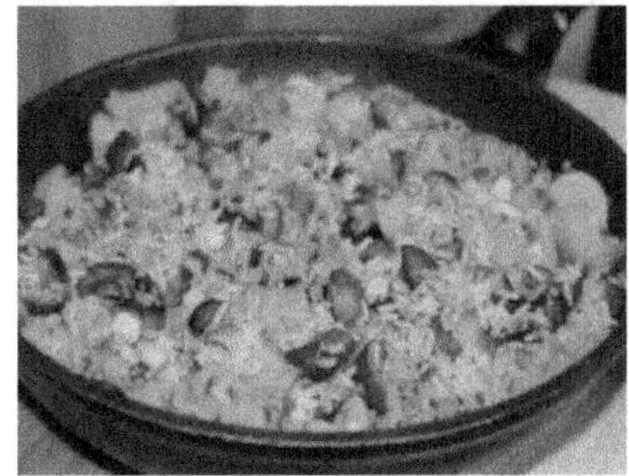

Ingredients:

For the Tofu-Carrots Mix:

½-block extra firm tofu, crumbled

2-tbsp reduced sodium soy sauce, gluten-free

½-cup onion, diced

1-cup carrot, diced

1-tsp turmeric

For the Cauliflower Cereal:

3-cups riced cauliflower

2-tbsp reduced sodium soy sauce, gluten-free

1½-tsp toasted sesame oil

1-tbsp rice vinegar

1-tbsp ginger, minced

½-cup broccoli, finely chopped

2-cloves garlic, minced

½-cup frozen peas

Directions:

1. Toss the tofu with the rest of the tofu-carrots mix ingredients. Place the mixture in your air fryer basket. Lock the lid, and set to cook for 10 minutes at 370°F.

2. Meanwhile, toss together all of the cauliflower cereal ingredients. Add this mixture to the air fryer pan. Lock the lid, and set to cook for another 10 minutes at 375°F.

Nutritional Values per Serving:

Calories: **390** | Fat: **32.6**g | Protein: **19.5**g | Total Carbohydrates: **17.4**g | Dietary Fiber: **12.7**g | Net Carbohydrates: **4.7**g

13-Stuffed Straw Mushroom Mobcap

Diet Specs: GF | VEG | NF

Yield: one serving

Serving Portion: 1-cup stuffed mushroom

Preparation Time: 15 minutes

Cooking Time: 5 minutes

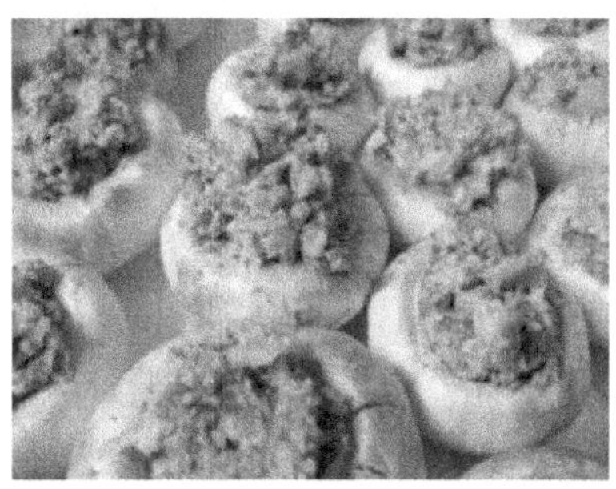

Ingredients:

1-cup fresh spinach, washed, bathed in ice, and drained

1-cup straw mushrooms or Chinese mushroom, washed and stems removed

1-tbsp coconut oil

1-bulb onion, finely chopped

1-clove garlic, minced

A dash of salt and pepper

A pinch of nutmeg

¼-cup quinoa, cooked

3.5-oz. cottage cheese

Directions:

1. Spread the spinach leaves over the food film while rolling them.

2. Fry the mushrooms with coconut oil in a saucepan before adding onion and garlic. Season the mushrooms with salt, pepper, and nutmeg. Set aside.

3. Combine the cooked quinoa with the cottage cheese. Spread the mixture evenly on the spinach leaves then roll into a pudding with the help of the food film.

4. Stuff the mushroom heads with the spinach pudding, and place them in the fridge.

5. Just before serving, slice the mushroom head with a sharp knife and pass quickly to the pan to heat.

Nutritional Values per Serving:

Calories: **401** | Fat: **34.7**g | Protein: **17.2**g | Total Carbohydrates: **16.9**g | Dietary Fiber: **11.4**g | Net Carbohydrates: **5**g

14-Crispy Chicken Packed in Pandan

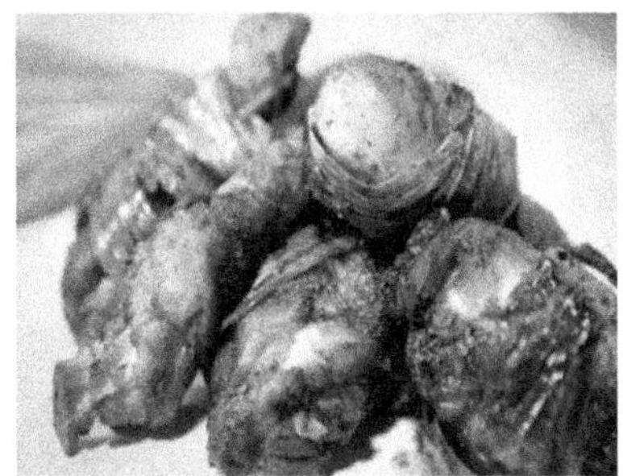

Diet Specs: GF | NF | DF

Yield: 4-servings

Serving Portion: 1 chicken thigh

Preparation Time: 30 minutes

Cooking Time: 18 minutes

Ingredients:

4-pcs (½-lb.) chicken thigh

1-tbsp shallot

1-pc lemon

1-tsp of fennel seeds

1-tsp of turmeric powder

1-tsp of chili powder

1-tbsp of oyster sauce, gluten-free

A pinch of salt

A pinch of sugar

A handful of pandan leaves

Directions:

1. Preheat your air fryer to 350°F for about 5 minutes.

2. Marinate the chicken with all the ingredients. Set aside for 30 minutes.

3. Wrap each chicken meat with the pandan leaves.

4. Arrange the wrapped chicken in the air fryer basket and lock the lid

5. Set to cook for 18 minutes at 375°F.

Nutritional Values per Serving:

Calories: **382** | Fat: **32.5**g | Protein: **17.8**g | Total Carbohydrates: **7.7**g | Dietary Fiber: **3.1**g | Net Carbohydrates: **4.6**g

15-Chicken Curry Masala Mix

Diet Specs: GF | NF | DF

Yield: 3-servings

Serving Portion: 1 serving bowl

Preparation Time: 10 minutes

Cooking Time: 35 minutes

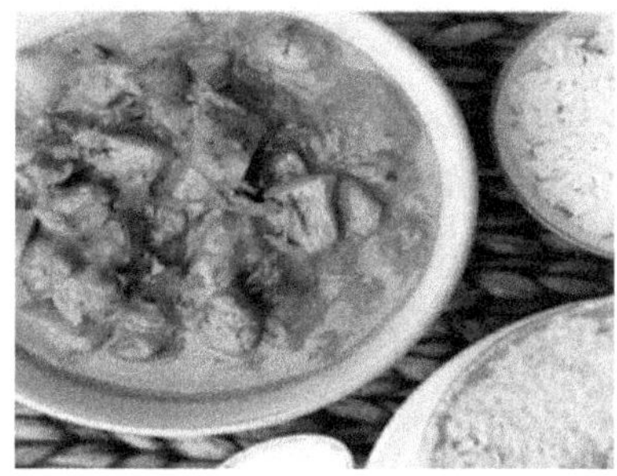

Ingredients:

2-tbsp sesame oil (divided)

2-tbsp ginger, diced

1½-lbs chicken thighs, boneless, skinless, and diced

1-cup tomatoes, chopped

¼-cup coriander, chopped

2-tsp turmeric

1-tsp cumin

1-tsp cayenne

2-tbsp lemon juice

Cilantro or mint leaves for garnish

Directions;

1. Sauté the ginger and jalapeno pepper with half of the sesame oil in a saucepan. Add the. Stir in the chicken, tomatoes, and coriander. Add the spices, the remaining sesame oil, lemon juice and half a cup of water.

2. Cover the saucepan, and cook for 30 minutes.

3. To serve, pour everything in a deep salad bowl, and garnish with cilantro or mint leaves.

Nutritional Values per Serving:

Calories: **377** | Fat: **29.3**g | Protein: **23.4**g | Total Carbohydrates: **6.8**g | Dietary Fiber: **1.9**g | Net Carbohydrates: **4.9**g

16-Milano Meatballs with Tangy Tomato

Diet Specs: GF | NF

Yield: 6-meatballs/3-servings

Serving Portion: 2 meatballs

Preparation Time: 25 minutes

Cooking Time: 30 minutes

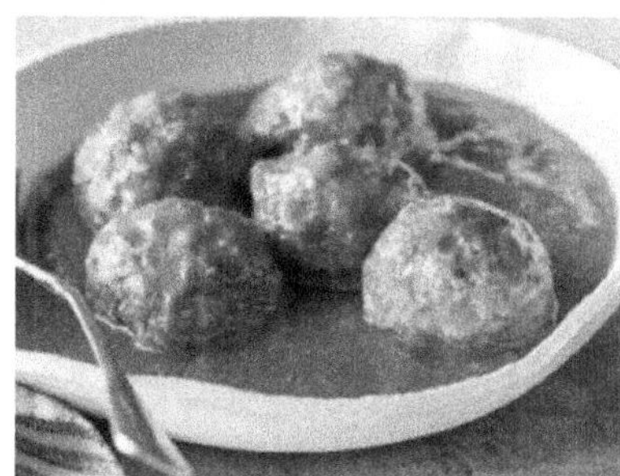

Ingredients:

For the Meatballs:

1-lb extra-lean ground beef

1-pc egg, whisked

10-pcs sun-dried tomatoes, chopped

½-cup ricotta cheese

1-cup Parmigiano-Reggiano cheese or parmesan cheese, freshly grated

A pinch of salt and freshly ground black pepper

For the Tomato Sauce:

1-bulb onion, finely chopped

¼-cup extra-virgin olive oil

2-lbs. tomato puree, gluten-free

A pinch of salt and freshly ground black pepper

Directions:

1. Combine all the meatball ingredients in a mixing bowl. Mix well until fully combined. Form balls from the mixture, and pat them down for even cooking.

2. Sauté the onions with olive oil in a skillet until they are translucent. Add the tomato puree and bring to a boil. Add the remaining ingredients and the meatballs. Cook for 30 minutes on medium heat.

TIP: For a vegetarian version of this recipe, you may replace the beef and pork meat with avocado and red potatoes.

Nutritional Values per Serving:

Calories: **396** | Fat: **32.6**g | Protein: **20.9**g | Total Carbohydrates: **8.2**g | Dietary Fiber: **3.4**g | Net Carbohydrates: **4.8**g

17-Aubergine À la Lasagna Lunch

Diet Specs: GF | VEG | NF

Yield: 2-lasagna sets/4-slices

Serving Portion: 1 lasagna slice

Preparation Time: 20 minutes

Cooking Time: 30 minutes

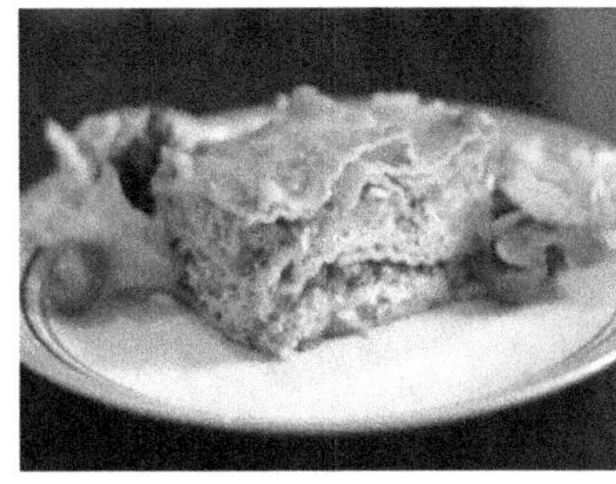

Ingredients:

2-pcs large eggplants, sliced and drained from excess liquid with a paper towel

A pinch of sea salt

2-cups part-skim ricotta cheese

½-cup parmesan cheese, freshly grated

1-pc egg, whisked

4-cups homemade tomato sauce, sugar-free

2-tbsp part-skim mozzarella cheese, shredded

2-tbsp cheddar cheese, grated

2-tbsp parsley, chopped

Directions:

1. Preheat your oven to 375°F. Meanwhile, season the eggplant slices with salt. Grill the eggplant slices for 3 minutes on each side.

2. Combine the ricotta, parmesan, and egg in a large bowl. Set aside.

3. Spread half of the tomato sauce in a saucepan. Layer half of the eggplant slices, and top with half of the cheddar and mozzarella. Pour half of the ricotta mixture over the layer, or just enough to coat it.

4. Cover the saucepan and insert into your preheated oven. Bake for 25 minutes. Set to cool for 10 minutes.

5. Repeat the process for the second lasagna set. To serve, garnish your lasagna with chopped parsley

Nutritional Values per Serving:

Calories: **346** | Fat: **27**g | Protein: **21.4**g | Total Carbohydrates: **7.9**g | Dietary Fiber: **3.5**g | Net Carbohydrates: **4.4**g

18-Beef Broccoli with Sesame Sauce

Diet Specs: GF | NF | DF

Yield: 4-servings

Serving Portion: 1 serving bowl

Preparation Time: 10 minutes

Cooking Time: 45 minutes

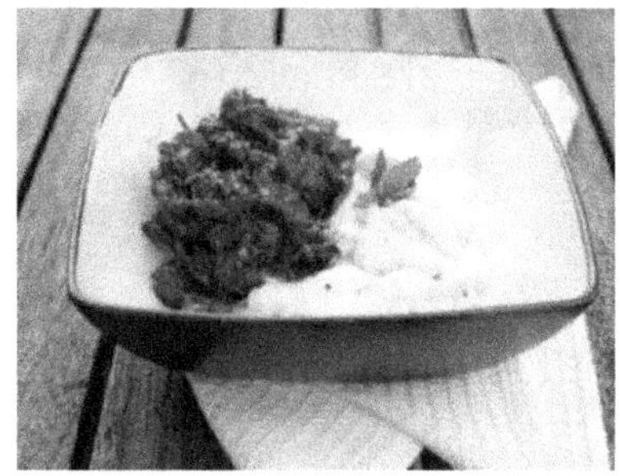

Ingredients:

2-tbsp coconut oil

1-tsp arrowroot powder

1-tbsp sesame oil

1-tbsp red fish sauce

½-tsp light sea salt

¼-tsp black pepper

¼-tsp baking powder

1-lb. beef, sliced into ¼-inch thick chunks

2-tsp sesame oil or olive oil

1-head broccoli, diced

2-tbsp coconut oil

2-cloves garlic, minced

2-ginger, finely chopped

A pinch of salt and pepper

Directions:

1. Mix the first seven ingredients in a bowl to make the sesame sauce. Set aside.

2. Fry the meat with sesame oil for 15 minutes until browned.

3. In a saucepan with water, add the broccoli, oil, garlic, and ginger. Season it with a pinch of salt and pepper. Add and spread the fried beef with the broccoli. Cover and cook for 20 minutes. Pour the sauce and cook for 10 more minutes.

Nutritional Values per Serving:

Calories: **375** | Fat: **31**g | Protein: **19.5**g | Total Carbohydrates: **5.4**g | Dietary Fiber: **0.8**g | Net Carbohydrates: **4.6**g

19- Sautéed Sirloin Steak in Sour Sauce

Diet Specs: NF

Yield: 4-servings

Serving Portion: 1 serving bowl

Preparation Time: 10 minutes

Cooking Time: 30 minutes

Ingredients:

1-bulb medium onion, chopped

1-clove garlic, minced

2-tbsp butter

1-lb. sirloin steak, trimmed and cut into thin strips

½-tsp salt

¼-tsp pepper

1-tbsp thyme

1½ cup fresh mushrooms, sliced

1-tbsp red wine vinegar

1-(10.5 oz.) can cream of mushroom soup

2-tbsp sour cream

4-cups egg noodles, cooked according to package instructions

Directions:

1. Sauté the onion and garlic with melted butter in a large skillet placed over medium heat. Remove from pan and set aside.

2. Add the beef strips, salt, pepper, and thyme. Cook evenly over low heat until browned.

3. Return the onion and garlic, and stir in the mushrooms, wine vinegar, and soup. Cover and simmer for 7 minutes until mushrooms are tender. Uncover and add sour cream. Stir and heat through. Serve immediately over the prepared noodles.

Nutritional Values per Serving:

Calories: **350** | Fat: **29.3**g | Protein: **17.7**g | Total Carbohydrates: **4.9**g | Dietary Fiber: **1**g | Net Carbohydrates: **3.9**g

20-Flaky Fillets with Garden Greens

Diet Specs: GF | NF | DF

Yield: 4-servings

Serving Portion: 1-fish fillet

Preparation Time: 25 minutes

Cooking Time: 30 minutes

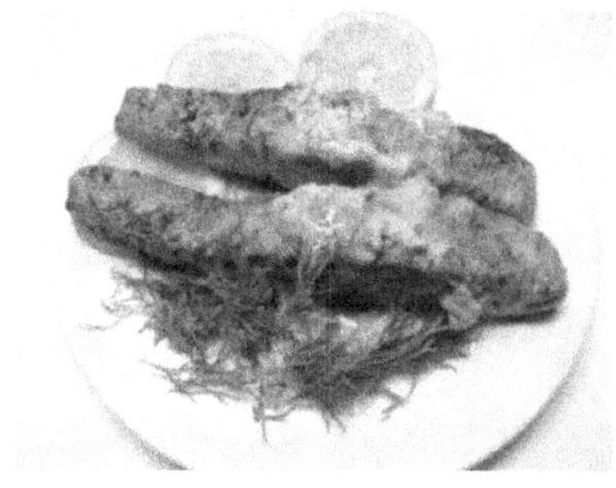

Ingredients:

1-lb broccoli, chopped into cubes and seasoned with a dash of salt and pepper

2-tbsp coconut oil

7-pcs scallions

2-tbsp small capers

1-tbsp sesame oil or olive oil

1½-lbs. white fish, sliced into 4 fillets

1-tbsp dried parsley

1¼-cups whipping cream, gluten-free and sugar-free

1-tbsp mustard, sugar-free

1-tsp of salt

¼-tsp ground black pepper

⅓-cup olive oil

5-oz.leafy greens

Directions:

1. Sauté the seasoned broccoli with sesame oil in a pan, and add the scallions and capers. Add the fish in the middle of the sautéed greens. Simmer for 15 minutes.

2. Meanwhile, mix the parsley with the whipping cream and mustard. Pour it over the cooked fish and vegetables. Drizzle with a little bit of coconut oil.

3. Return the saucepan on medium heat and cook for an extra 10 minutes.

Nutritional Values per Serving:

Calories: **395** | Fat: **33**g | Protein: **19.8**g | Total Carbohydrates: **8.7**g | Dietary Fiber: **3.9**g | Net Carbohydrates: **4.8**g

Chapter 7-Dinner Delights

1-Pizza Pie with Cheesy Cauliflower Crust

Diet Specs: GF | VEG | NF

Yield: 4-pizza wedges/2-servings

Serving Portion: 2-pizza wedges

Preparation Time: 5 minutes

Cooking Time: 30 minutes

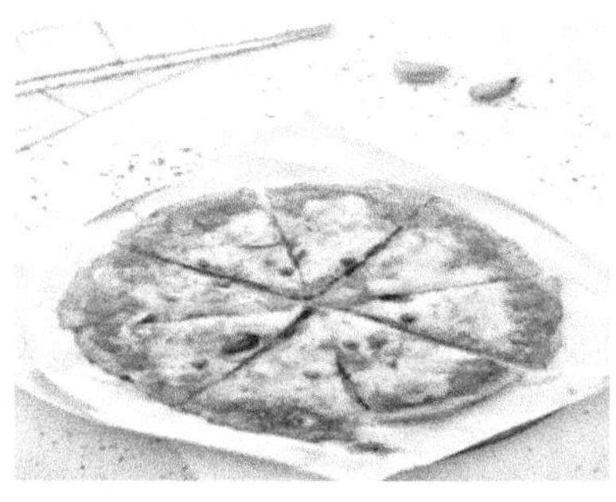

Ingredients:

½-head cauliflower, rinsed, riced, cooked for 5 minutes in boiling water, and drained

2-pcs eggs, whisked

⅓-parmesan cheese

½-cup cherry tomatoes, washed and halved

2-tbsp organic hempseed oil

1-tsp balsamic vinegar

1-mozzarella cheese ball, crumbled

¼-cup basil leaves

Directions:

1. Spin the cooked cauliflower in a dishtowel to let out as much liquid as possible. (The goal is to obtain a flour texture.) Add the eggs and cheese. Mix well.

2. Spread to a disk the cauliflower dough on a baking pan lined with parchment paper. Bake for 15 minutes at 400°F in your preheated oven.

3. Meanwhile, mix the tomatoes with hempseed oil and balsamic vinegar. Season the mixture with salt and pepper.

4. Remove the pizza dough from the oven. Add the tomato mixture and sprinkle over with mozzarella. Return the pan in the oven and bake further for 15 minutes.

5. Serve hot and garnish with fresh basil leaves.

Nutritional Values per Serving:

Calories: **384** | Fat: **32.1**g | Protein: **19.9**g | Total Carbohydrates: **5.5**g | Dietary Fiber: **1.7**g | Net Carbohydrates: **3.8**g

2-Roasted Rib-eye Skillet Steak

Diet Specs: GF | NF

Yield: 2-servings

Serving Portion: 1 slice rib-eye steak

Preparation Time: 5 minutes

Cooking Time: 15 minutes

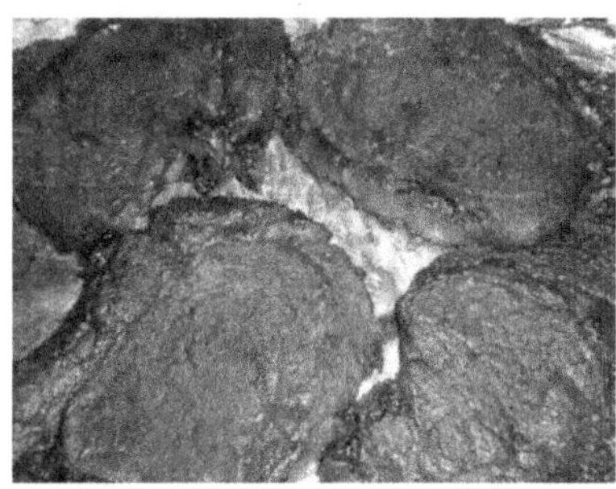

Ingredients:

1-16oz rib-eye steak (1 to 1¼-inch thick)

2-tbsp duck fat or peanut oil (divided)

A dash of salt and pepper

1-tbsp butter

½-tsp thyme, chopped

Directions:

1. Preheat your oven to 400°F. Place a cast iron skillet inside.

2. Season the rib-eye steak with oil, salt, and pepper.

3. Take the preheated skillet out from the oven and place over the stove, set in medium heat. Pour oil, and add the steak. Sear for 2 minutes on both sides.

4. Return the skillet with the steak in the oven. Roast for 6 minutes.

5. Remove the skillet and place over the stove, set in low heat. Add the butter and thyme in the skillet. Baste the steak for about 4 minutes.

Nutritional Values per Serving:

Calories: **722** | Fat: **60.2**g | Protein: **45**g | Total Carbohydrates: **0**g | Dietary Fiber: **0**g | Net Carbohydrates: **0**g

3-À la Spaghetti with Asian Sauce

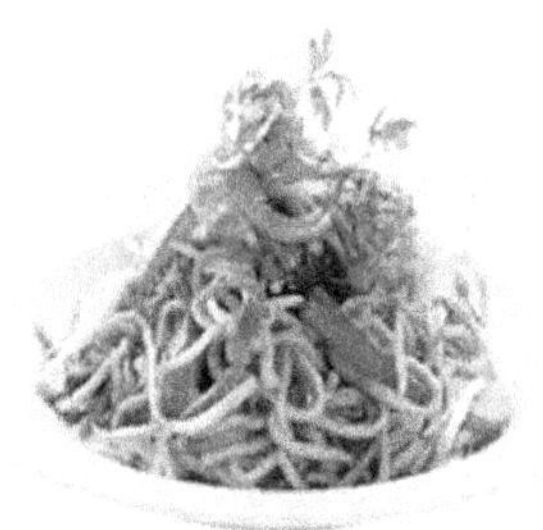

Diet Specs: GF | VEG | DF

Yield: 2-servings

Serving Portion: 1 serving plate

Preparation Time: 10 minutes

Cooking Time: 15 minutes

Ingredients:

For the Sauce:

2-tbsp soy sauce, gluten-free

1-tsp of hemp oil

1-tsp of lemon juice

1-tbsp peanut butter

For the Spaghetti:

½-bulb onion, diced

1-tsp coconut oil

1-tsp red or green pepper, diced

1-pc carrot, thinly sliced lengthwise

1 egg, whisked

5-oz. low-carb spaghetti, rinsed and cooked for 2 minutes in boiling water

Fresh coriander and peanuts for garnish

Directions:

1. Combine all the sauce ingredients in a bowl. Set aside.

2. Sauté the onion with oil, and add the peppers, carrots, egg, sauce, and spaghetti. Cook for 13 minutes, stirring frequently.

3. To serve, garnish with fresh coriander and peanuts.

Nutritional Values per Serving:

Calories: **412** | Fat: **34.4**g | Protein: **20.9**g | Total Carbohydrates: **10.5**g | Dietary Fiber: **5.7**g | Net Carbohydrates: **4.8**g

4-Shirataki & Soy Sprouts Pad Thai with Peanut Tidbits

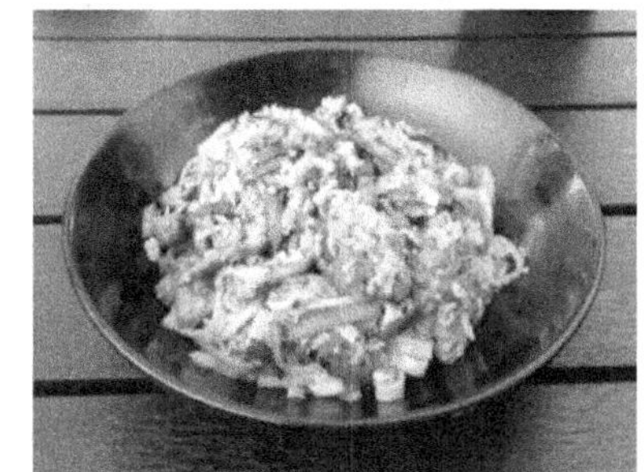

Diet Specs: GF | VEG | DF

Yield: one serving

Serving Portion: 1 serving bowl

Preparation Time: 10 minutes

Cooking Time: 5 minutes

Ingredients:

For the Sauce:

1-tbsp peanut butter

2-tbsp soy sauce, gluten-free

½-lime

2-tbsp agave syrup, gluten-free

½-tbsp organic turmeric

For the Noodles:

1-bag of konjac shirataki noodles, rinsed and cooked for 2 minutes in boiling water

1-pc carrot, thinly sliced

1-bulb onion, thinly sliced

½-cup soy sprouts

¼-cup unsalted peanuts

Some sprigs of fresh coriander

Directions:

1. Combine all the sauce ingredients in a bowl. Set aside.

2. Heat the pasta with a little coconut oil in a frying pan. Pour the sauce and add the coriander. Mix well and cook for 5 minutes.

3. To serve, place in a bowl and garnish with peanuts and coriander sprigs.

Nutritional Values per Serving:

Calories: **423** | Fat: **35.2**g | Protein: **21**g | Total Carbohydrates: **14.9**g | Dietary Fiber: **9.6**g | Net Carbohydrates: **5.3**g

5-Charred Chicken with Squash Seed Sauce

Diet Specs: NF | DF

Yield: 2-chicken skewers/one serving

Serving Portion: 2-chicken skewers

Preparation Time: 15 minutes

Cooking Time: 20 minutes

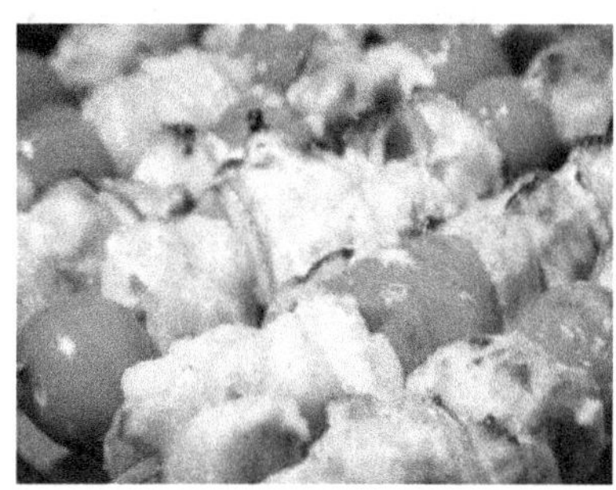

Ingredients:

For the Sauce:

2-tbsp white almond puree

2-cloves of garlic, finely chopped (divided, for the sauce and chicken marinade)

½-tbsp squash seeds

1-tbsp barley

1-pc fresh basil

For the Marinade:

2-branches rosemary, finely chopped

1-pc red chili, finely chopped

1-pc lemon (keep the zest)

Pinch of salt and ground black pepper

1-tbsp olive oil

1-cup chicken breasts, cubed

5-bulbs small onions, sliced in quarters

5-pcs cherry tomatoes

Directions:

1. Combine and mix all the sauce ingredients in a bowl. Set aside.

2. Mix all the marinade ingredients and let stand for 10 minutes. Thread alternately the onions, meat, and tomatoes into the skewers and grill over coal fire for 10 minutes on each side. Serve the chicken kebabs with the squash seed sauce.

Nutritional Values per Serving:

Calories: **428** | Fat: **35.6**g | Protein: **21**g | Total Carbohydrates: **16.9**g | Dietary Fiber: **11.6**g | Net Carbohydrates: **5.3**g

6-Therapeutic Turmeric & Shirataki Soup

Diet Specs: NF | DF

Yield: one serving

Serving Portion: 1 serving bowl

Preparation Time: 10 minutes

Cooking Time: 32 minutes

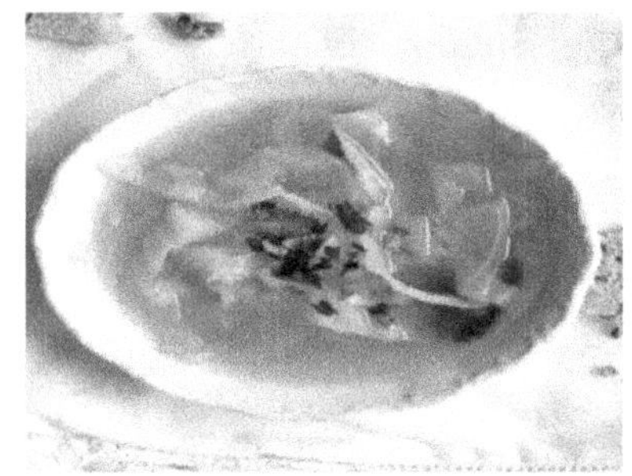

Ingredients:

1-tbsp turmeric powder

1-serving chicken-vegetable broth soup

3-pcs carrots, sliced into small pieces

3-slices ginger

1-pack (5-oz.) konjac shirataki noodles

¼-lb. chicken breast, sliced into strips

Directions:

1. Simmer all the ingredients over low heat for 30 minutes.

2. Rinse the konjac noodles thoroughly under cold water.

3. Add the noodles to the broth and heat for 2 minutes.

TIP: This is a great therapeutic dish when acquiring keto flu.

Nutritional Values per Serving:

Calories: **415** | Fat: **34.6**g | Protein: **21.6**g | Total Carbohydrates: **10.1**g | Dietary Fiber: **5.7**g | Net Carbohydrates: **4.4**g

7-Fresh Fettuccine with Pumpkin Pesto

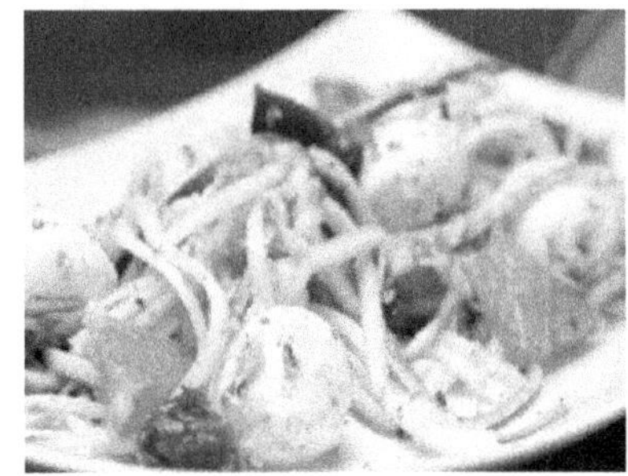

Diet Specs: VEG | NF

Yield: 3-servings

Serving Portion: 1 serving bowl

Preparation Time: 15 minutes

Cooking Time: 2 minutes

Ingredients:

For the Pesto Sauce:

1-tbsp olive oil

1-tbsp pumpkin seed oil

½-tsp pumpkin seeds

¼-cup barley

1-tbsp lemon juice

A pinch salt

For the Pasta:

1¾-cup zucchini, washed, peeled, and cut into thin noodle strips

½-cup cherry tomatoes, washed and cut in half

1¼-cup low carb fettuccine

1-pc mozzarella cheeseball

A pinch of pepper

Directions:

1. Combine and mix all the sauce ingredients with 2-tbsp water in a bowl. Set aside.

2. Boil the fettuccine for 1 minute and add the zucchini. Boil further for another minute, and drain.

3. Toss the pasta with the pesto sauce. Season the dish with a pinch of pepper and garnish with tomatoes and mozzarella.

Nutritional Values per Serving:

Calories: **417** | Fat: **34.7**g | Protein: **20.9**g | Total Carbohydrates: **10.5**g | Dietary Fiber: **5.3**g | Net Carbohydrates: **5.2**g

8- Cheddar Chicken Casserole

Diet Specs: GF | NF

Yield: 6-servings

Serving Portion: 1 serving plate

Preparation Time: 10 minutes

Cooking Time: 30 minutes

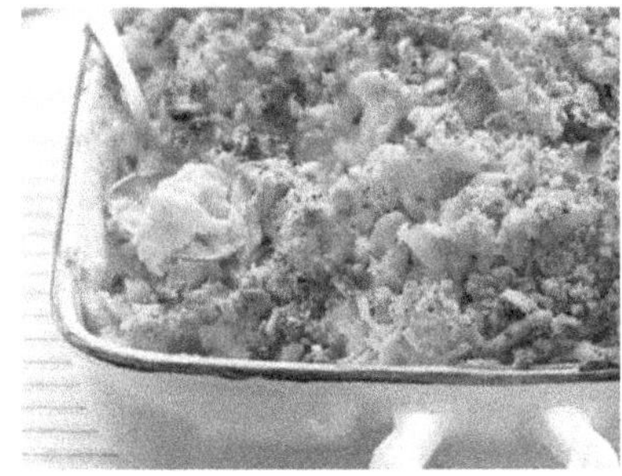

Ingredients:

20-oz. chicken breasts

2-tbsp olive oil (divided)

2-cups broccoli, steamed

½-cup sour cream

½-cup heavy cream

1-oz. pork rinds, crushed

A dash of salt and pepper

½-tsp paprika

1-tsp oregano

1-cup cheddar cheese, grated

Directions:

1. Preheat your oven to 450°F.

2. Sear the chicken with a tablespoon of olive oil in a pan until it cooks all the way through. Shred the meat in the pan. Add the remaining oil, broccoli, and sour cream.

3. Place and spread evenly the mixture in an 8" x11" pan. Press firmly and drizzle with heavy cream. Add all the remaining seasonings and top the casserole with the cheese. Place the pan in the oven and bake for 25 minutes until the edges turn brown and start bubbling.

Nutritional Values per Serving:

Calories: **405** | Fat: **33.8**g | Protein: **22.7**g | Total Carbohydrates: **3.6**g | Dietary Fiber: **1**g | Net Carbohydrates: **2.6**g

9-Zesty Zucchini Pseudo Pasta & Sweet Spanish Onions Overload

Diet Specs: VEG | NF | DF

Yield: 2-servings

Serving Portion: 1 serving bowl

Preparation Time: 10 minutes

Cooking Time: 20 minutes

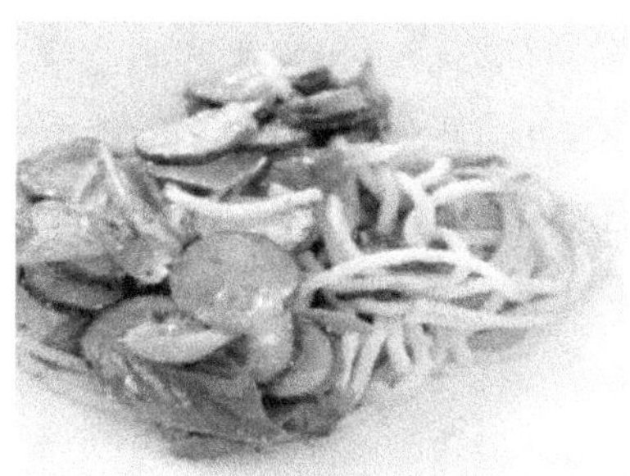

Ingredients:

2-tbsp of vegetable oil

2-pcs yellow onions or Spanish onions

1-tbsp low-sodium soy sauce

2-tbsp low-sodium teriyaki sauce

1-tbsp sesame seeds

4-pcs small zucchinis, sliced into spaghetti strips using a spiral cutter

Directions:

1. Add the vegetable oil, onions, and soy sauce to a saucepan placed over medium heat. Stir in the teriyaki sauce and sesame seeds. Mix well until fully combined.

2. Cook for 10 minutes, stirring frequently until the vegetables turn brown.

3. Add the zucchini pasta and cook for 3 minutes.

4. To serve, transfer the pasta in a serving dish and garnish with chopped parsley.

Nutritional Values per Serving:

Calories: **319** | Fat: **25.9**g | Protein: **18.1**g | Total Carbohydrates: **6.6**g | Dietary Fiber: **3.2**g | Net Carbohydrates: **3.4**g

10-Soba & Spinach Sprouts

Diet Specs: GF | VEG | DF

Yield: 2-servings

Serving Portion: 1 serving bowl

Preparation Time: 15 minutes

Cooking Time: 0 minutes

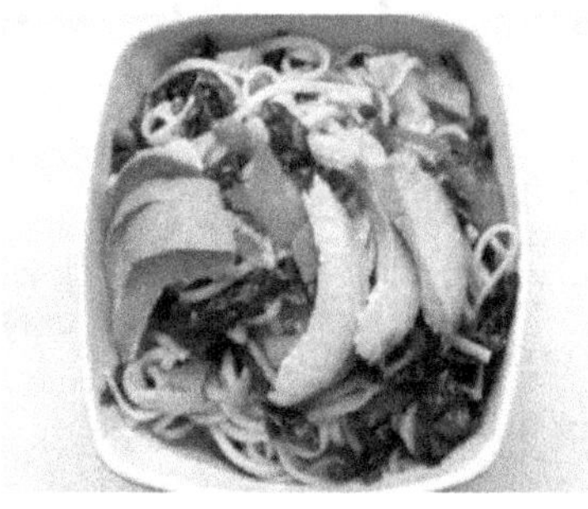

Ingredients:

3-pcs mushrooms, sliced into quarters

⅓-cup smoked tofu, sliced into squares

1-tbsp coconut oil

½-pc green pepper, sliced into strips

3-tbsp cashew nuts

½- clove garlic

½-pc lime, juice

A dash of salt and pepper

¼-cup water (more, as needed)

¼-cup soba noodles, cooked according to package instructions

1⅓-cup spinach sprouts

1-tbsp coconut shavings for garnish

Directions:

1. Fry the mushrooms and tofu with coconut oil in a frying pan until they turn brown. Add the pepper. Set aside.

2. For the sauce, mix cashews with garlic, lime juice, salt, pepper, and a little water.

3. Divide the noodles between two bowls and top with spinach sprouts. Arrange the remaining vegetables on top. Garnish with coconut shavings or avocado slices, sesame seeds, and a slice of lime.

4. To serve, pour over the sauce on each arranged bowl.

Nutritional Values per Serving:

Calories: **355** | Fat: **29.6**g | Protein: **17.8**g | Total Carbohydrates: **8.3**g | Dietary Fiber: **3.9**g | Net Carbohydrates: **4.4**g

11-Chickpeas & Carrot Consommé

Diet Specs: GF | VEG | NF | DF

Yield: 2-servings

Serving Portion: 1 serving bowl

Preparation Time: 10 minutes

Cooking Time: 20 minutes

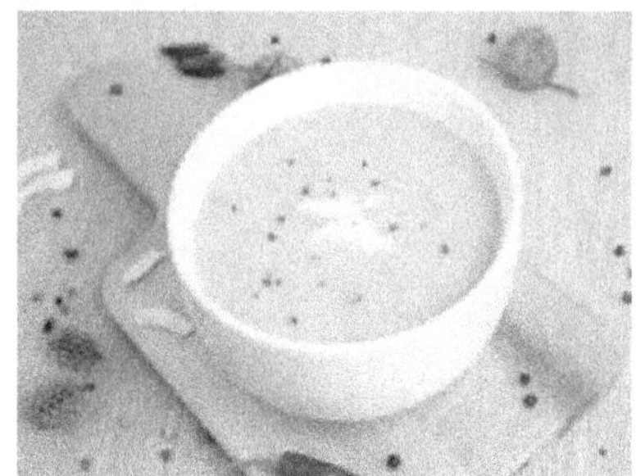

Ingredients:

¼-lb. chickpeas, cooked

1-tbsp coconut oil

1-clove garlic, minced

1-piece ginger, minced

1-bulb small onion, finely chopped

½-lb. carrots, sliced into small pieces

1¼-cup vegetable broth

A dash of salt and pepper

½-cup coconut milk

1-tbsp coconut shaving

Directions:

1. Arrange the chickpeas on a plate lined with parchment paper. Sprinkle with salt, curry, and paprika. Spread the spices well and bake for 15 minutes at 350°F.

2. Melt the coconut oil in a saucepan and brown the garlic, ginger, and onion. Add the carrots. Deglaze with vegetable broth and simmer for 15 minutes over medium heat until the carrots cook through.

3. Season to taste with salt, pepper, curry, and paprika. Pour the coconut milk.

4. Mix the soup and garnish with chickpeas and coconut shavings.

TIP: This soup will also be delicious with sweet potatoes, potatoes, parsnip, beetroot, spinach, mushrooms, broccoli, peas, tofu, chicken, coriander or parsley.

Nutritional Values per Serving:

Calories: **460** | Fat: **38.2**g | Protein: **23.3**g | Total Carbohydrates: **10.1**g | Dietary Fiber: **4.3**g | Net Carbohydrates: **5.8**g

12-Chicken Cauliflower Curry

Diet Specs: GF | NF | DF

Yield: 2-servings

Serving Portion: 1 serving bowl

Preparation Time: 15 minutes

Cooking Time: 30 minutes

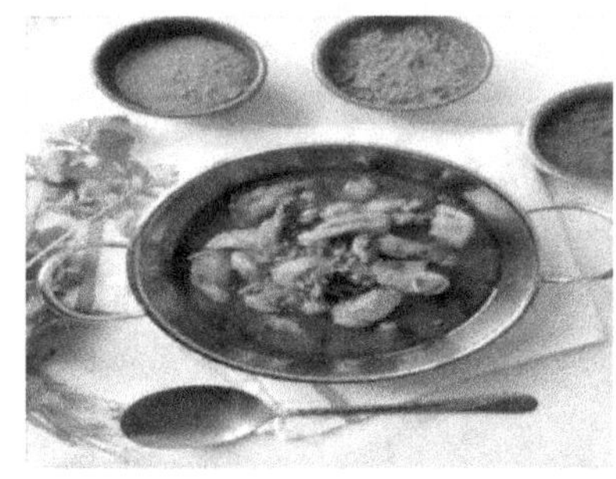

Ingredients

1-cup vegetable broth

1-tbsp curry paste

½-cup light coconut milk

½-lb chicken breast, cooked and sliced into small pieces

1-pc potato, diced

1-clove garlic, minced

½-bulb onion, finely chopped

1-cup cauliflower, diced

⅓-cup fresh peas

Salt and pepper

¼-cup goji berries

Directions:

1. Heat the vegetable broth in a wok for 5 minutes. Add the curry paste, coconut milk, meat, potato, garlic, and onion. Cook for 15 minutes.

2. Add the vegetables and cook further for 10 minutes until they are tender. Season the curry with a dash of salt and pepper.

3. To serve, garnish with goji berries.

TIP: If the sauce reduces too quickly, it is possible to add broth.

Nutritional Values per Serving:

Calories: **334** | Fat: **27**g | Protein: **18.7**g | Total Carbohydrates: **8.4**g |
Dietary Fiber: **4.3**g | Net Carbohydrates: **4.1**g

13-Cheesy Cauliflower Mac Munchies

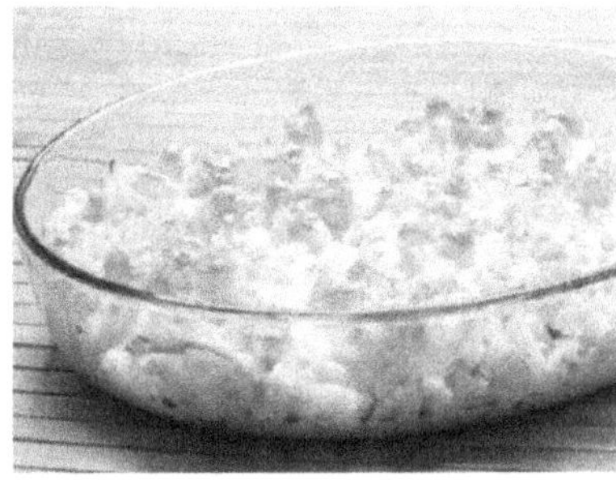

Diet Specs: GF | VEG

Yield: 2-servings

Serving Portion: 1 serving bowl

Preparation Time: 20 minutes

Cooking Time: 15 minutes

Ingredients:

1-pc medium cauliflower, riced

3-tbsp + ½-tsp avocado oil (divided)

A pinch of sea salt

A pinch of black pepper

1-cup cheddar cheese, shredded

¼-cup cream, gluten-free

¼-cup almond milk, unsweetened

Directions:

1. Preheat your air fryer to 400°F. Spray the pan with oil.

2. Place the riced cauliflower in the pan and drizzle with the avocado oil. Toss well and season with a pinch each of salt and pepper. Set aside.

3. Heat the cheese, cream, and milk with a little bit of avocado oil in a pot.

4. Pour the cheese mixture over the seasoned cauliflower. Lock the lid of the air fryer and set to cook for 14 minutes.

Nutritional Values per Serving:

Calories: **352** | Fat: **27.8**g | Protein: **20.9**g | Total Carbohydrates: **8.9**g | Dietary Fiber: **4.3**g | Net Carbohydrates: **4.6**g

14-Sugar Snap Pea Pods with Coco Crunch

Diet Specs: GF | VEG | NF | DF

Yield: 2-servings

Serving Portion: 1 serving bowl

Preparation Time: 5 minutes

Cooking Time: 10 minutes

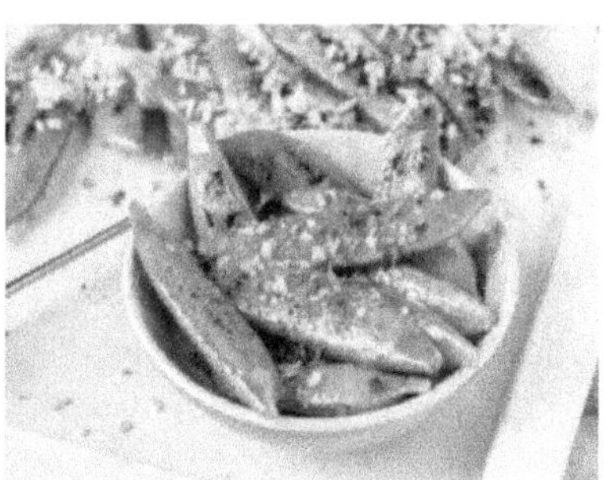

Ingredients:

4-tbsp salted butter, gluten-free and dairy-free

1-tbsp coconut oil

½-cup coconut, unsweetened and shredded

⅛-tsp cinnamon

1-tbsp rosemary oil

9-oz. snap pea pods, trimmed, strings removed, and diced

A pinch of salt

Directions:

1. In a saucepan, melt the coconut oil with the butter over medium heat. Add the coconut shreds, rosemary oil, and cinnamon. Toss very well until fully incorporated.

2. Add the diced pea pods and mix again. Leave to cook for 8 minutes until the pea pods start to melt.

3. To serve, sprinkle over a pinch of salt.

Nutritional Values per Serving:

Calories: **389** | Fat: **31.3**g | Protein: **22**g | Total Carbohydrates: **7.2**g | Dietary Fiber: **2.3**g | Net Carbohydrates: **4.9**g

15-Spicy & Smoky Spinach-Set Fish Fillets

Diet Specs: GF | NF | DF

Yield: 2-servings

Serving Portion: 1-fish fillet

Preparation Time: 15 minutes

Cooking Time: 10 minutes

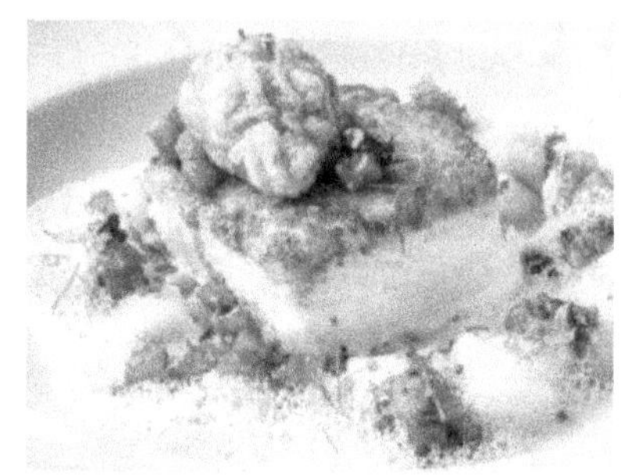

Ingredients:

2-pcs halibut meat (11-oz. each), membrane removed and deboned

4-cups packed spinach

Juice of ½-pc lemon

A pinch of salt and pepper

A pinch of smoked paprika

1-pc sliced lemon

1-pc green onions, sliced

1-pc red chili, deseeded and thinly sliced

1-cup cherry tomatoes, halved

2-tbsp avocado oil

Directions:

1. Place the halibut meat over a flat surface. Divide the spinach between them.

2. Lay each halibut meat on each pile of spinach. Squeeze the lemon over each part and season with smoked paprika.

3. Top each fish meat with lemon slices, green onions, chili, and the cherry tomatoes. Pour 1-tbsp of avocado oil over each fish portion.

4. Wrap around each fish meat tightly with foil; arrange them in a baking pan. Cook for 10 mins until the fish turns golden and flaky when forked.

TIP: You can use sesame or coconut oil instead of avocado oil and use salmon instead of halibut.

Nutritional Values per Serving:

Calories: **248** | Fat: **18.8**g | Protein: **15.3**g | Total Carbohydrates: **13.2**g | Dietary Fiber: **8.9**g | Net Carbohydrates: **4.3**g

16-Spicy Shrimps & Sweet Shishito

Diet Specs: GF | NF | DF

Yield: 2-servings

Serving Portion: 1 serving bowl

Preparation Time: 15 minutes

Cooking Time: 15 minutes

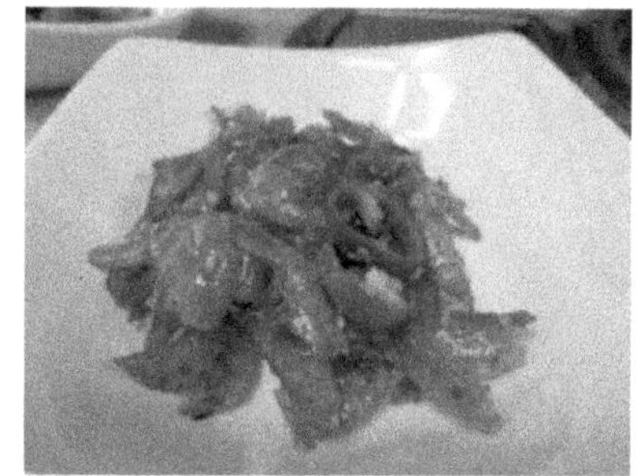

Ingredients:

2-tbsp canola oil

A pinch of sea salt

1-clove garlic, crushed and finely chopped

1-pc red chili pepper, seeded and finely chopped

5-oz. whole shishito peppers

10-oz. shrimps, jumbo size

1-tsp sesame oil

2-tbsp low-sodium light soy sauce

Juice of 1-pc lime

Directions:

1. Preheat your air fryer to 350°F for about 5 minutes. Spray your air fryer pan with canola oil.

2. Add the salt, garlic, and red chili pepper. Mix well until fully combined.

3. Add the shishito peppers; mix thoroughly again. Add the shrimps and drizzle with sesame oil.

4. Place the pan in your air fryer and lock the lid. Cook for about 10 minutes at 400°F

5. Divide the dish equally between three serving bowls. To serve, season each bowl with lime juice and soy sauce.

Nutritional Values per Serving:

Calories: **370** | Fat: **28.9**g | Protein: **23**g | Total Carbohydrates: **7.2**g | Dietary Fiber: **2.8**g | Net Carbohydrates: **4.4**g

17-Spaghetti-Styled Zesty Zucchini with Guacamole Garnish

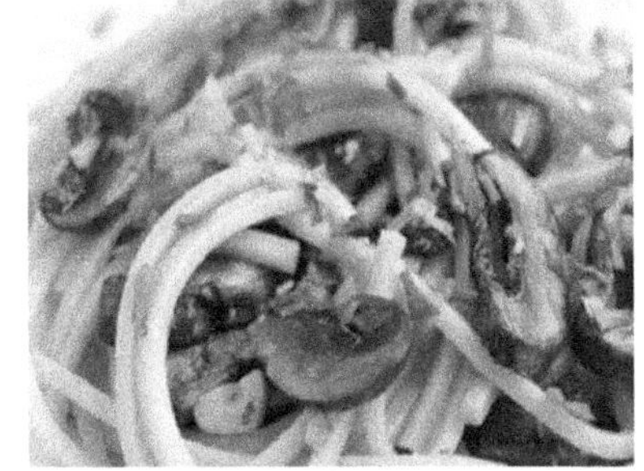

Diet Specs: GF | VEG | NF | DF

Yield: 2-servings

Serving Portion: 1-set of guacamole and carbonara

Preparation Time: 15 minutes

Cooking Time: 5 minutes

Ingredients:

2-pcs medium zucchini, cut into spaghetti strips using a spiral cutter

1-tbsp sea salt

1-pc large avocado, peeled, pitted, and cut into small pieces

1⅓-cup fresh basil, washed, dried and finely chopped

2-tbsp lemon juice

A dash of salt and black pepper

1-tbsp coconut oil

7-oz. mushrooms, cleaned and cut into slices

1-pc pomegranate, seeds extracted

Directions:

1. Season the zucchini strips with sea salt and set aside.

2. Mix the avocado slices, lemon juice, and a dash of salt and pepper. Set aside.

3. Toss lightly the zucchini in a frying pan placed over medium heat. Fry for 4 to 5 minutes in coconut oil. Add the mushrooms and pomegranate seeds.

4. To serve, place the zucchini spaghetti on a plate with the avocado cream in a separate bowl. Garnish with the basil leaves.

TIP: To peel quickly and cleanly a pomegranate, cut the fruit in half, and hold a half over a bowl or plate. Gently tap the back of the fruit with a tablespoon so that the beans come out. Scrape the most persistent grains directly with the spoon.

Nutritional Values per Serving:

Calories: **381** | Fat: **31.8**g | Protein: **19**g | Total Carbohydrates: **14.3**g | Dietary Fiber: **9.5**g | Net Carbohydrates: **4.8**g

18-Grain-less Gnocchi in Melted Mozzarella

Diet Specs: GF | VEG | NF

Yield: one serving

Serving Portion: 1 serving bowl

Preparation Time: 10 minutes

Cooking Time: 15 minutes

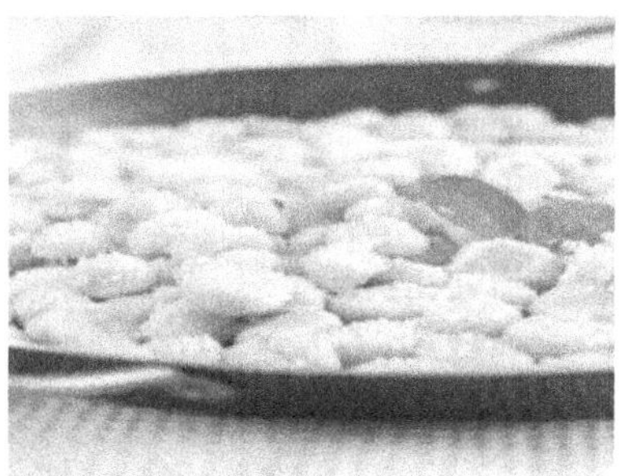

Ingredients:

2-cups mozzarella, shredded

½-tsp garlic powder

1-tsp salt

3-pcs large egg yolks, whisked (divided)

½-cup tomato sauce, gluten-free

Directions:

1. Melt the mozzarella with the garlic powder and salt for 5 minutes in a microwave-safe dish.

2. Pour half of the egg yolks into the mozzarella mixture in a large bowl. Mix until fully combined. Add the remaining egg yolks. Mix thoroughly again until fully incorporated.

3. Divide the mixture into four parts. Roll each part into a long rope over a flat surface. Cut each rope into gnocchi-like pieces, pressing each with a fork.

4. Bring a pan filled with water to a boil. Add the gnocchi dumplings and cook for about 2 minutes.

5. Preheat your air fryer to 350°F. Spray the air fryer pan with cooking oil.

6. Arrange the gnocchi pieces in the air fryer pan. Lock the lid of the air fryer and cook for 10 minutes.

7. To serve, pour the tomato sauce over the gnocchi.

Nutritional Values per Serving:

Calories: **355** | Fat: **27.6**g | Protein: **22.1**g | Total Carbohydrates: **6.5**g | Dietary Fiber: **2.1**g | Net Carbohydrates: **4.4**g

19-Cauliflower Chao Fan Fried with Pork Pastiche

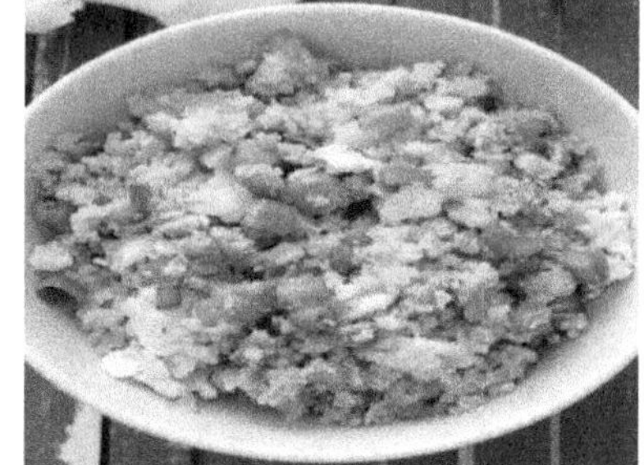

Diet Specs: GF | NF | DF

Yield: 4-servings

Serving Portion: 1 serving bowl

Preparation Time: 20 minutes

Cooking Time: 15 minutes

Ingredients:

½-head medium-sized cauliflower, chopped into small cubes

2-pcs eggs

2-cloves garlic, chopped

2-cups pork belly, cut into thin strips

3-pcs green capsicums

2-bulbs onions

1-tbsp soy sauce, gluten-free

1-tsp black sesame seeds

1-tbsp spring onion, chopped

1-tsp pickled ginger

Directions:

1. Place the chopped cauliflower in your food processor; pulse into smaller granules. Set aside.

2. Whisk the eggs, and swirl in the frying pan. Cook for 3 minutes.

3. Add the pork belly strips and the cauliflower rice. Stir in the onions and soy sauce. Cook for about 10 minutes.

4. To serve, distribute the preparation equally between four serving bowls. Garnish with sesame seeds, spring onions, and pickled ginger.

Nutritional Values per Serving:

Calories: **460** | Fat: **35.7**g | Protein: **28.6**g | Total Carbohydrates: **8.3**g | Dietary Fiber: **2.3**g | Net Carbohydrates: **6**g

20-All-Avocado Stuffed with Spicy Beef Bits

Diet Specs: GF | NF

Yield: 6-servings

Serving Portion: 1-halved avocado

Preparation Time: 20 minutes

Cooking Time: 20 minutes

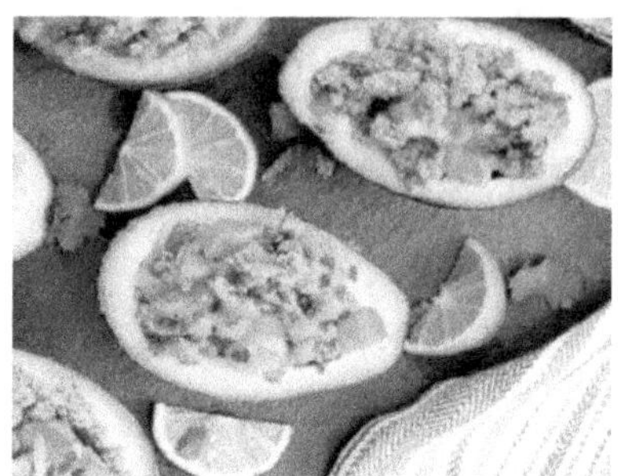

Ingredients:

1-lb. ground beef

1-tbsp chili powder

½-tsp salt

¾-tsp cumin

½-tsp dried oregano

¼-tsp garlic powder

¼-tsp onion powder

4-oz. tomato sauce, gluten-free

3-pcs medium-sized avocados, halved and pitted

1-cup cheddar cheese, shredded for garnish

¼-cup cherry tomatoes, sliced for garnish

¼-cup lettuce, shredded for garnish

A dash of chopped cilantro for garnish

Directions:

1. Cook the beef with oil and a little water in a pan for 10 minutes, stirring frequently until it turns brown. Stir in the spices and tomato sauce. Cook for another 10 minutes.

2. Load the cooked beef to each halved avocado and top with garnish.

Nutritional Values per Serving:

Calories: **280** | Fat: **23.1**g | Protein: **14**g | Total Carbohydrates: **6.3**g | Dietary Fiber: **2.2**g | Net Carbohydrates: **4.1**g

Chapter 8-Satisfying Snacks

1-Coconut Candy

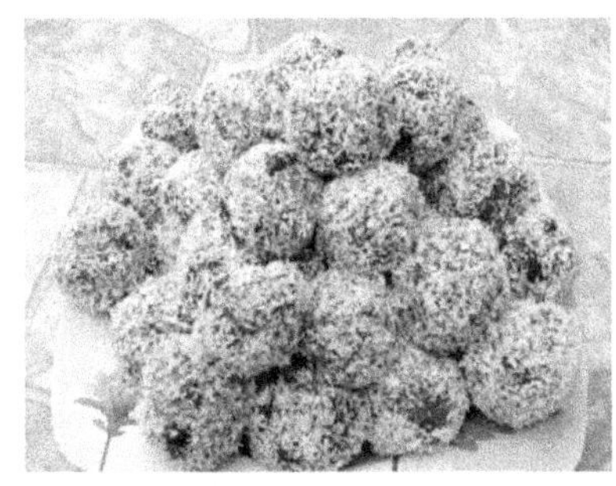

Diet Specs: GF | VEG | NF | DF

Yield: 4-candy balls/1-serving

Serving Portion: 4-candy balls

Preparation Time: 10 minutes

Cooking Time: 0 minutes

Ingredients:

2-tbsp coconut butter (or notably known as Coconut Manna)

Directions:

1. Melt the coconut butter at room temperature until it resembles a creamy butter consistency.

2. Spoon out the melted butter into candy molds. Refrigerate for 10 minutes to harden before serving.

TIP: You can make more candies and refrigerate it for several weeks placed in a closed container.

Nutritional Values per Serving:

Calories: **204** | Fat: **17.2**g | Protein: **10.2**g | Total Carbohydrates: **3**g | Dietary Fiber: **0.8**g | Net Carbohydrates: **2.2**g

2-Mozzarella Mound Munchies

Diet Specs: VEG | NF

Yield: 3-servings

Serving Portion: 1-mozzarella cheese mound

Preparation Time: 5 minutes

Cooking Time: 6 minutes

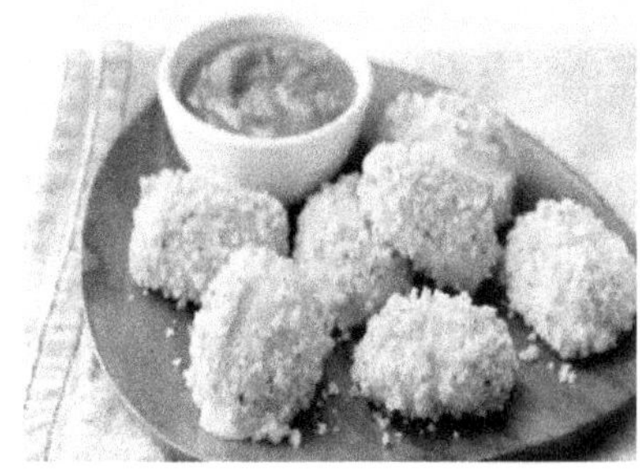

Ingredients:

⅓-cup panko bread, herb-flavored

2-pcs egg whites

6-tbsp mozzarella cheese, molded into 2-tbsp balls

¼-cup marinara sauce

Directions:

1. Preheat your oven to 425°F.

2. Toast the panko breadcrumbs for 2 minutes, stirring frequently, in a medium skillet placed over medium heat.

3. Transfer the breadcrumbs in a bowl. Add the egg whites into a separate bowl.

4. Dip a cheeseball into the egg and roll in the panko. Place the breaded cheese on a greased baking sheet, and bake for 3 minutes. Repeat the process for the remaining cheese.

5. Heat the marinara sauce in your microwave oven for half a minute. Serve the breaded cheeseball with the sauce

Nutritional Values per Serving:

Calories: **157** | Fat: **13.2**g | Protein: **5.9**g | Total Carbohydrates: **4.8**g | Dietary Fiber: **1.1**g | Net Carbohydrates: **3.7**g

3-Philadelphia Potato Praline

Diet Specs: GF | VEG | NF

Yield: 8 x 45-calorie pralines /2-servings

Serving Portion: 4-pralines

Preparation Time: 30 minutes

Cooking Time: 0 minutes

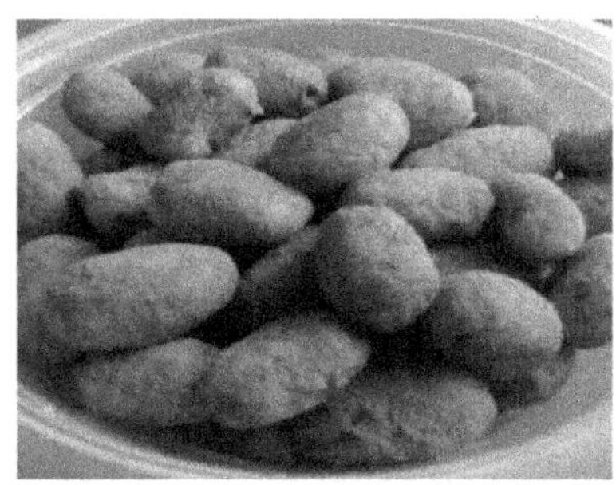

Ingredients:

⅓-cup Philadelphia cream cheese

1½-cup coconut, unsweetened and shredded

1-tbsp butter

¼-tsp ground cinnamon

Sweetener of choice

Directions:

1. Combine all the ingredients except for the ground cinnamon in a bowl. Refrigerate the mixture and allow setting until it hardens.

2. Divide the mixture into 8 portions and roll each portion into potato shapes. Place them on a sheet of parchment paper.

3. Sprinkle all over with the cinnamon and store in the fridge for a week before serving.

TIP: When making more servings, apportion the batter by its weight by summing up the total weight of the ingredients less the cinnamon, and dividing by the number of servings desired.

Nutritional Values per Serving:

Calories: **180** | Fat: **15.3**g | Protein: **8.9**g | Total Carbohydrates: **3.2**g | Dietary Fiber: **1.5**g | Net Carbohydrates: **1.7**g

4-Tasty Turkey Cheese Cylinders

Diet Specs: GF | NF

Yield: one serving

Serving Portion: 2-rollups

Preparation Time: 5 minutes

Cooking Time: 0 minutes

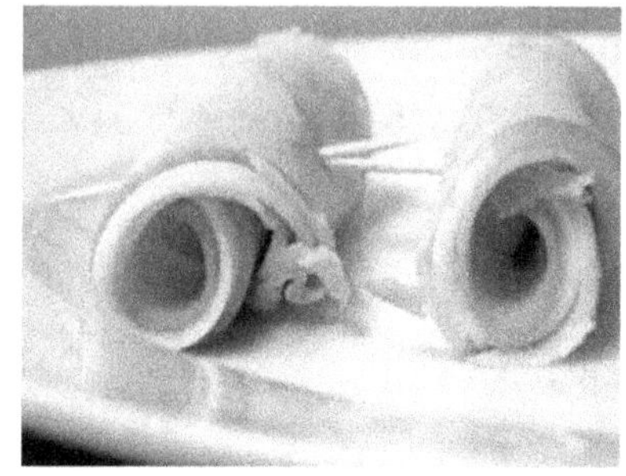

Ingredients:

1-oz. turkey, roasted and sliced

1-oz. cheese

Directions:

1. Slice the cheese into a long strip, enough to fit the turkey slice.

2. Wrap the turkey slice around the cheese.

Nutritional Values per Serving:

Calories: **162** | Fat: **10.9**g | Protein: **15.6**g | Total Carbohydrates: **3.8**g | Dietary Fiber: **0**g | Net Carbohydrates: **3.8**g

5-Fried Flaxseed Tortilla Treat

Diet Specs: VEG | NF | DF

Yield: 3-servings

Serving Portion: 2-shells flaxseed tortillas

Preparation Time: 5 minutes

Cooking Time: 10 minutes

Ingredients:

6-shells flaxseed tortillas, sliced into chip-sized cuts

3-tbsp olive oil

A dash of salt and pepper

Directions:

1. Fry the flaxseed chips with olive oil in a large pan placed over medium-high heat. Cook for 10 minutes until the chips become crispy, stirring frequently. Strain the chips and place on a paper towel to drain excess oil.

2. Season the chips with a dash of salt and pepper.

Nutritional Values per Serving:

Calories: **36** | Fat: **2.8**g | Protein: **0.8**g | Total Carbohydrates: **2.7**g | Dietary Fiber: **0.7**g | Net Carbohydrates: **2**g

6-Power-Packed Butter Balls

Diet Specs: GF | VEG | DF

Yield: 10-balls/5-servings

Serving Portion: 2-butter balls

Preparation Time: 80 minutes

Cooking Time: 0 minutes

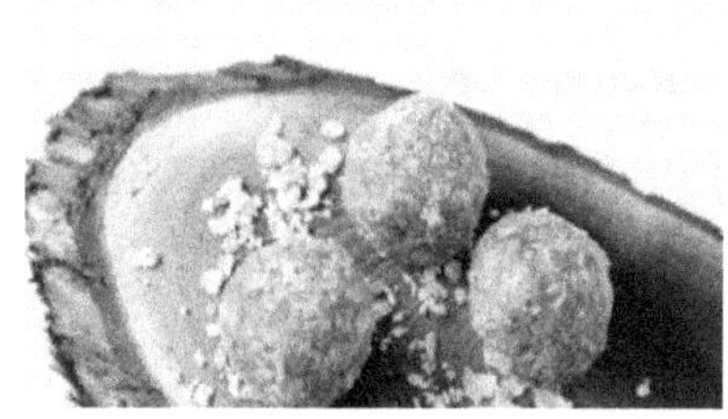

Ingredients:

2-tbsp cocoa powder + 1-tbsp for dusting

2-tbsp plain oatmeal, gluten-free

⅔-cup peanut butter or chia butter

1-tbsp organic chia seeds

3-tbsp protein powder

Directions:

1. Mix the cocoa powder, oatmeal, peanut butter chia seeds, and protein powder.

2. By using your hand, form balls from the mixture. Dust each ball with cocoa powder.

3. Place the balls in the fridge for 1 hour before serving.

Nutritional Values per Serving:

Calories: **128** | Fat: **10.1**g | Protein: **4.9**g | Total Carbohydrates: **7.2**g | Dietary Fiber: **2.9**g | Net Carbohydrates: **4.3**g

7-Choco Coco Cups

Diet Specs: GF | VEG | NF | DF

Yield: 20-mini cups/10-servings

Serving Portion: 2-mini cups

Preparation Time: 50 minutes

Cooking Time: 0 minutes

Ingredients:

For the Coconut Base:

½-cup coconut butter

½-cup coconut oil

½-cup unsweetened coconut, shredded

3-tbsp powdered sweetener

For the Chocolate Topping:

3-oz. sugar-free dark chocolate

Directions:

1. Line a muffin pan with 20 mini parchment cups.

2. Heat the coconut butter with the coconut oil in a saucepan placed over low heat. Stir until the butter melts. Stir in the shredded coconut and sweetener until fully combined.

3. Divide the mixture equally between the prepared muffin cups. Freeze for 30 minutes until firm.

4. Melt the dark chocolate and spoon over the cold filling. Let it set for 15 minutes before serving.

TIP: You can store the candy cups in your countertop for up to a week.

Nutritional Values per Serving:

Calories: **240** | Fat: **25.3**g | Protein: **2.1**g | Total Carbohydrates: **5**g | Dietary Fiber: **4**g | Net Carbohydrates: **1**g

8-Corndog Clumps

Diet Specs: GF

Yield: 20-corndogs/10-servings

Serving Portion: 2-corndogs

Preparation Time: 5 minutes

Cooking Time: 15 minutes

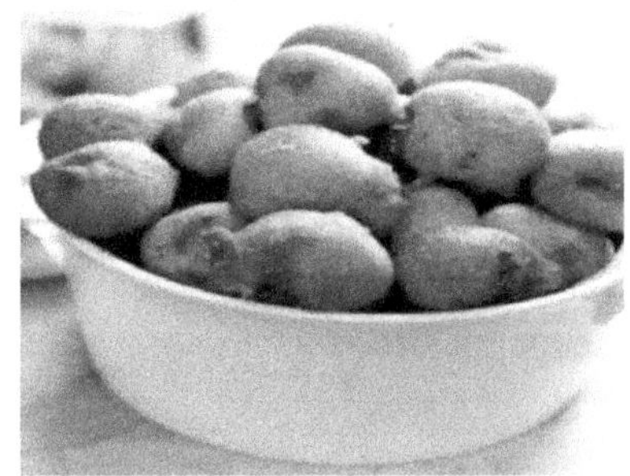

Ingredients:

¼-tsp. baking powder

¼-tsp. salt

½-cup almond flour

½-cup flaxseed meal

1-tbsp psyllium husk powder

3-packets sweetener

1-pc large egg

⅓-cup sour cream

¼-cup melted butter

¼-cup coconut milk

10-pcs (2-oz.) smoked sausage, sliced in half

Directions:

1. Preheat your oven to 375°F. Grease a 20-cup muffin pan.

2. Combine the first six ingredients in a bowl. Add the egg, sour cream, and butter and mix well. Pour in the coconut milk, and mix again. Pour the batter in the pan.

3. Insert a sliced sausage into the center of each muffin. Place the pan in the oven.

4. Bake for 12 minutes; thereafter, broil for 3 minutes, set on high heat.

Nutritional Values per Serving:

Calories: **148** | Fat: **13.2**g | Protein: **3.9**g | Total Carbohydrates: **4**g | Dietary Fiber: **1.6**g | Net Carbohydrates: **3.4**g

9-Kingly Kale Crispy Chips

Diet Specs: GF | V | NF | DF

Yield: one -serving

Serving Portion: 1 serving bowl

Preparation Time: 0 minutes

Cooking Time: 0 minutes

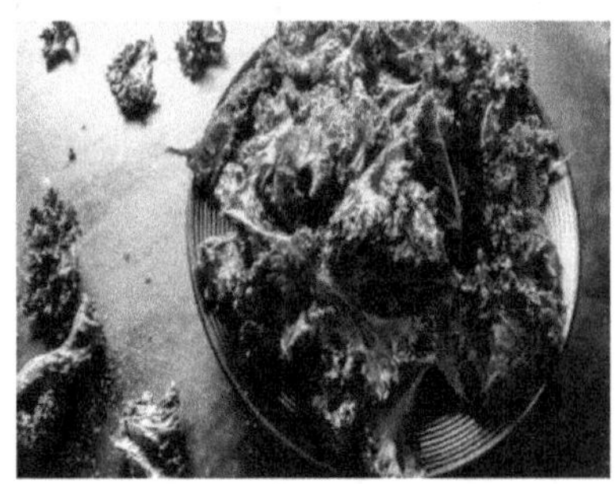

Ingredients

1-bunch large kale, rinsed, drained, and stemless

2-tbsp olive oil

1-tbsp salt

Directions:

1. Preheat your oven to 350°F.

2. Place the kale in a plastic bag. Pour the oil, and mix well by shaking the bag until coating thoroughly each leaf.

3. Spread the kale onto a baking sheet. Press the leaves flat to obtain an evenly crisped cook for each leaf.

4. Bake for 12 minutes until the edges turn brown while the rest of the kales remain dark green.

5. Sprinkle the salt over the baked kale and serve.

TIP: There is a fine line between perfect baking and overcooking the kale leaves. Overcooked kale comes out with a very bitter taste.

Nutritional Values per Serving:

Calories: **81** | Fat: **7.6**g | Protein: **1.9**g | Total Carbohydrates: **2.1**g | Dietary Fiber: **0.9**g | Net Carbohydrates: **1.2**g

10-Ambrosial Avocado Puree Pudding

Diet Specs: GF | VEG | NF | DF

Yield: 3-servings

Serving Portion: 1-glass

Preparation Time: 5 minutes

Cooking Time: 0 minutes

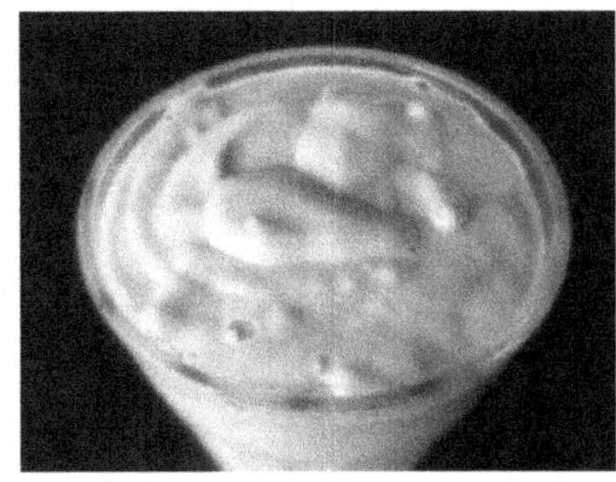

Ingredients

2-ripe Hass avocados, peeled, pitted and cut into chunks

2-tsp organic vanilla extract

80-drops of liquid sweetener

1-can (113.5-oz.) organic coconut milk

1-tbsp lime juice from organic lime

Directions

1. Combine all the ingredients in a blender. Blend to a smooth and velvety consistency. Pour the blend equally between three glasses. Chill before serving.

Nutritional Values per Serving:

Calories: **240** | Fat: **23.8**g | Protein: **2.8**g | Total Carbohydrates: **12.8**g | Dietary Fiber: **9**g | Net Carbohydrates: **3.8**g

Chapter 9-Delectable Desserts

1-Cool Cucumber Sushi with Sriracha Sauce

Diet Specs: GF | VEG | NF | DF

Yield: 12-cucumber sushi slices/4-servings

Serving Portion: 3-cucumber sushi slices

Preparation Time: 20 minutes

Cooking Time: 0 minutes

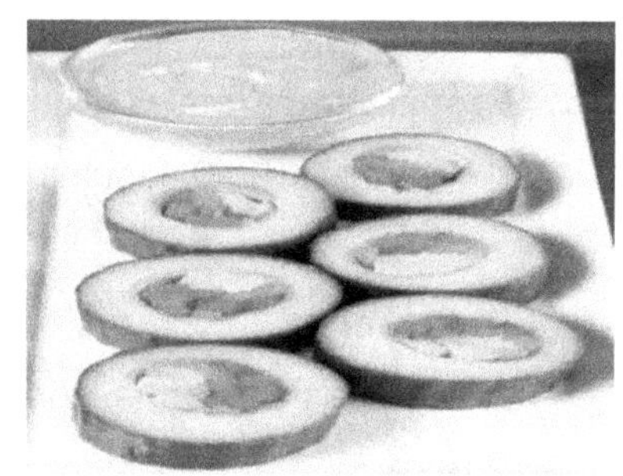

Ingredients:

For the Sushi:

2-pcs medium cucumbers

¼-pc avocado, thinly sliced

2-pcs small carrots, thinly sliced

½-pc red bell pepper, thinly sliced

½-pc yellow bell pepper, thinly sliced

For the Sriracha Sauce:

⅓-cup mayonnaise

1-tbsp sriracha

1-tsp soy sauce, gluten-free

Directions:

1. Slice one end of the cucumbers, and core them by using a small spoon to remove the seeds until completely hollow.

2. By using a butter knife, press the avocado slices into the center of each cucumber. Slide in the carrots and bell peppers until filling up completely each cucumber.

3. To make the dipping sauce, whisk to combine all the sauce ingredients in a bowl.

4. Slice the cucumber into 1"-thick round pieces, Serve with sauce on the side.

Nutritional Values per Serving:

Calories: **110** | Fat: **10.1**g | Protein: **1.9**g | Total Carbohydrates: **4.8**g | Dietary Fiber: **2**g | Net Carbohydrates: **2.8**g

2-Coco Crack Bake-less Biscuit Bars

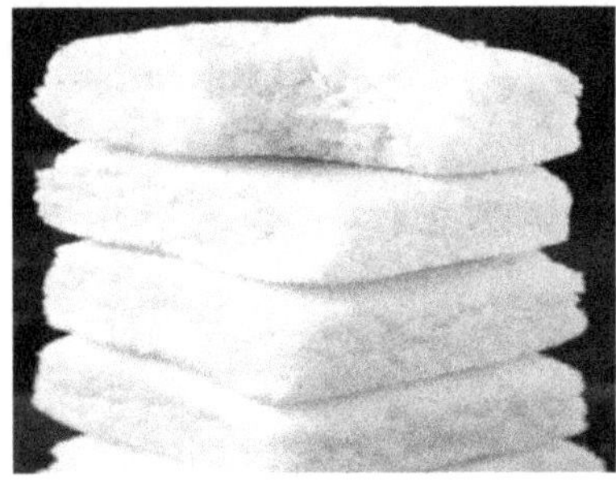

Diet Specs: GF | V | NF | DF

Yield: 20-servings

Serving Portion: 1-bar

Preparation Time: 2 minutes

Cooking Time: 3 minutes

Ingredients:

3-cups unsweetened coconut flakes, shredded

1-cup coconut oil, melted

¼-cup liquid sweetener of choice

Directions:

1. Line an 8"-square baking pan with parchment paper. Set aside.

2. Combine all the ingredients in a large mixing bowl. Mix well to a thick batter. (Add a little liquid sweetener or water if the batter is too crumbly.

3. Pour and press firmly the mixture in the prepared pan. Refrigerate until firm.

4. To serve, slice the hardened mixture into 2" x 8" bars.

TIP: You can store the bars in covered jars at room temperature (covered) for up to a week; up to a month when refrigerated; and, up to a couple of months when frozen.

Nutritional Values per Serving:

Calories: **106** | Fat: **10.5**g | Protein: **2.9**g | Total Carbohydrates: **2**g | Dietary Fiber: **2**g | Net Carbohydrates: **0**g

3-Chocolate-Coated Sweet Strawberries

Diet Specs: GF | V | NF | DF

Yield: 16-candy cubes/8-servings

Serving Portion: 2-candy cubes

Preparation Time: 4 hours 10 minutes

Cooking Time: 0 minutes

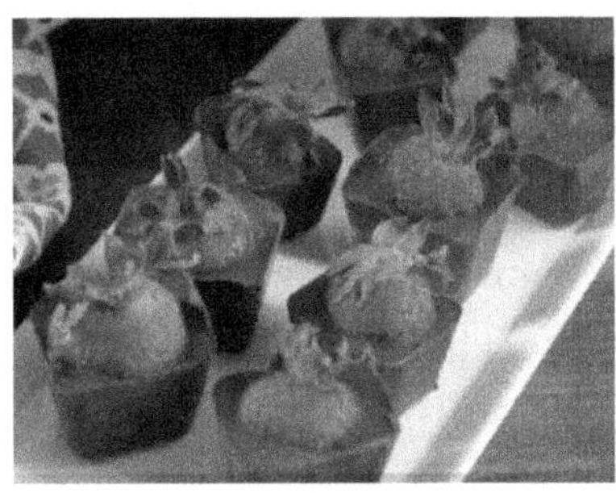

Ingredients:

2-cups melted chocolate chips, dairy-free

2-tbsp coconut oil

16-pcs fresh strawberries, with stems

Directions:

1. Combine the melted chocolate and coconut oil in a medium bowl. Mix well until fully combined.

2. Scoop the chocolate mixture into each mold of an ice cube tray. Top each with a strawberry, with its stem part up. Pour the remaining chocolate mixture over strawberries. Freeze for 4 hours until the chocolate hardens.

Nutritional Values per Serving:

Calories: **125** | Fat: **11.1**g | Protein: **2.7**g | Total Carbohydrates: **5**g | Dietary Fiber: **1.4**g | Net Carbohydrates: **3.6**g

4-Matcha Muffins with Choco-Coco Coating

Diet Specs: GF | VEG | DF

Yield: 8-muffins/4-servings

Serving Portion: 2-muffins

Preparation Time: 15 minutes

Cooking Time: 15 minutes

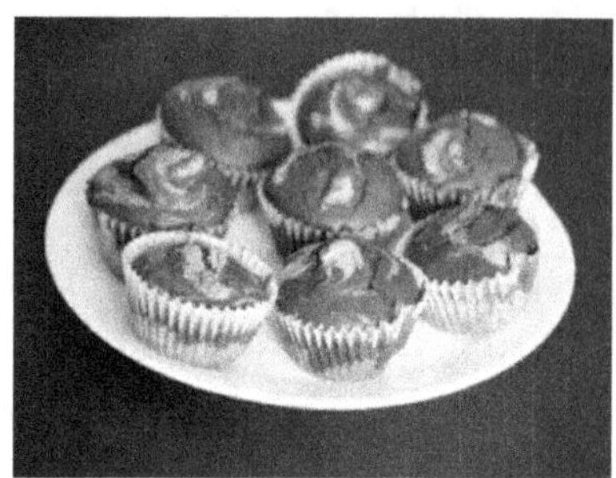

Ingredients:

½-cup almond flour

1-tbsp yeast

1-tbsp cooking matcha powder

1-tbsp cashew nuts

½-cup milk substitute with hydrogenated vegetable oil

1-tbsp peanut butter

1-tbsp cacao nibs

1-tbsp coconut syrup, gluten-free

3-tbsp milk substitute with hydrogenated vegetable oil

A handful of Goji berries (or blueberries and raspberries) and cocoa nuggets (optional)

Directions:

1. Mix the flour, yeast, matcha powder, cashews. Pour ½-cup of vegetable milk gradually while mixing into dough.

2. Put dough in a pre-greased muffin pan. Bake for 15 minutes at 350°F.

3. Mix the peanut butter with cacao, syrup, and milk to make the icing. To serve, pour the icing and garnish with cocoa nuggets and Goji berries.

Nutritional Values per Serving:

Calories: **140** | Fat: **10.9**g | Protein: **5.1**g | Total Carbohydrates: **8.8**g | Dietary Fiber: **3.4**g | Net Carbohydrates: **5.4**g

5-Cinnamon Cup Cake

Diet Specs: GF | V | NF | DF

Yield: one serving

Serving Portion: 1-cup cake

Preparation Time: 1 minute

Cooking Time: 0 minutes

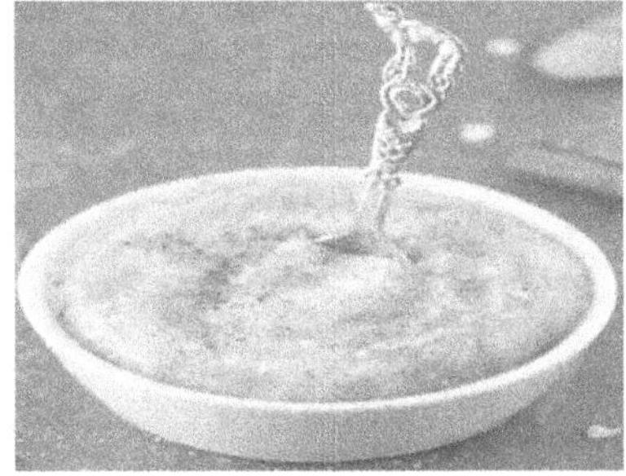

Ingredients:

1-scoop vanilla protein powder

½-tsp baking powder

1-tbsp coconut flour

½-tsp cinnamon

1-tbsp granulated sweetener of choice

¼-cup almond milk

¼-tsp vanilla extract

1-tsp granulated sweetener of choice

½-tsp cinnamon powder

For the Butter Glaze:

1-tbsp coconut butter, melted

½-tsp almond milk

A pinch of cinnamon powder

Directions:

1. Combine the protein powder, baking powder, coconut flour, cinnamon, and sweetener in a greased microwave-safe bowl. Mix well until fully combined.

2. Pour the milk, vanilla extract, and sweetener. Mix thoroughly to form a batter. (Add a little milk if the batter is too crumbly). Top with a sprinkling of cinnamon powder.

3. Cook in the microwave for 1-minute. Meanwhile, combine all the butter glaze ingredients in a bowl. To serve, top the cake with the butter glaze.

Nutritional Values per Serving:

Calories: **263** | Fat: **24.1**g | Protein: **7.6**g | Total Carbohydrates: **14.2**g | Dietary Fiber: **10.3**g | Net Carbohydrates: **3.9**g

6-Choco 'Cado Twin Truffles

Diet Specs: GF | V | NF | DF

Yield: 15-candy balls/5-servings

Serving Portion: 3-candy balls

Preparation Time: 30 minutes

Cooking Time: 0 minutes

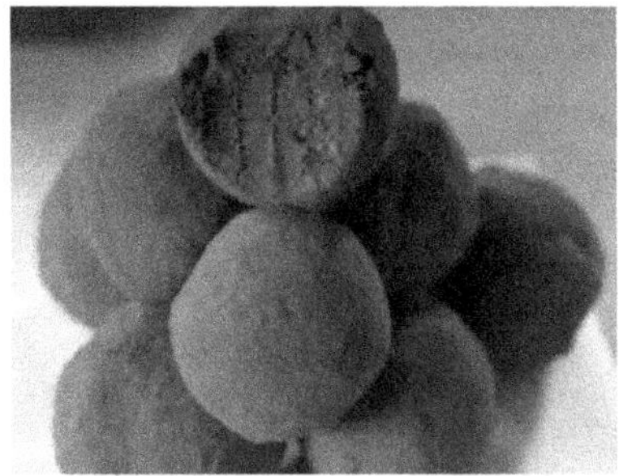

Ingredients:

1-cup melted dark chocolate chips, dairy-free

1-pc small avocado, mashed

1-tsp vanilla extract

¼-tsp kosher salt

¼-cup cocoa powder

Directions:

1. Combine the melted chocolate with avocado, vanilla, and salt in a bowl. Mix well until fully combined. Refrigerate for 20 minutes to firm up slightly.

2. By using a small spoon, scoop about a tablespoon of the chocolate mixture and roll it in the palm of your hand to form a ball. Repeat the process to consume the mixture.

3. Roll each ball in cocoa powder.

Nutritional Values per Serving:

Calories: **68** | Fat: **5.8**g | Protein: **1.6**g | Total Carbohydrates: **4.2**g | Dietary Fiber: **1.8**g | Net Carbohydrates: **2.4**g

7-Butter Ball Bombs

Diet Specs: GF | V | DF

Yield: 30-servings/10-servings

Serving Portion: 3-butter balls

Preparation Time: 65mins

Cooking Time: 0 minutes

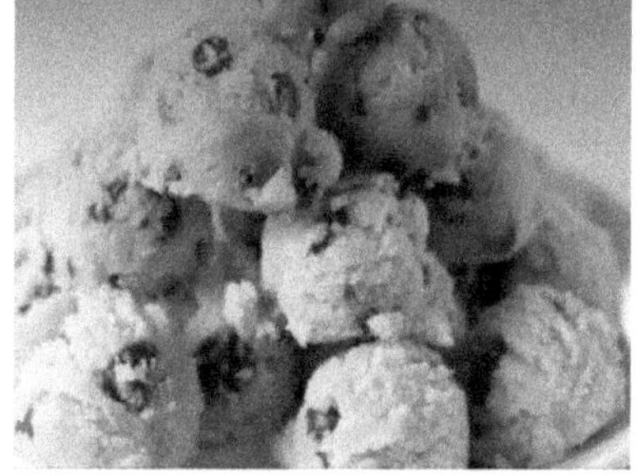

Ingredients:

8-tbsp (1 stick) butter, softened to room temperature

⅓-cup sweetener

½-tsp. pure vanilla extract

½-tsp. kosher salt

2-cups almond flour

⅔-cup unsweetened dark chocolate chips, dairy-free

Directions:

1. By using your hand mixer, beat the butter in a large bowl until light and fluffy. Add the sweetener, vanilla extract, and salt. Beat again until fully combined.

2. Add gradually the almond flour, beating continuously until no dry portions remain. Fold in the chocolate chips. Cover the bowl with a plastic wrap and refrigerate for 20 minutes to firm slightly.

3. By using a small spoon, scoop the dough to form into small balls.

TIP: You can store the balls for up to a week inside the fridge and up to a month inside the freezer.

Nutritional Values per Serving:

Calories: **51** | Fat: **4.3**g | Protein: **0.7**g | Total Carbohydrates: **2.7**g | Dietary Fiber: **0.4**g | Net Carbohydrates: **2.3**g

8-Choco Coco Cookies

Diet Specs: GF | VEG

Yield: 18-servings/6-servings

Serving Portion: 3-cookies

Preparation Time: 10 minutes

Cooking Time: 15 minutes

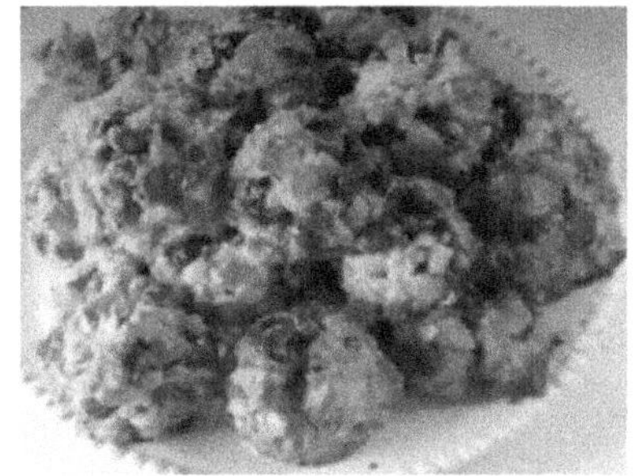

Ingredients:

¼-cup coconut oil

4-tbsp butter, softened

2-tbsp sweetener

4-pcs egg yolks

1-cup dark unsweetened chocolate chips

1-cup coconut flakes

¾-cup roughly chopped walnuts

Directions:

1. Preheat your oven to 350°F. Line a baking tray with parchment paper.

2. Combine all the ingredients in a large mixing bowl stir together coconut oil, butter, sweetener, and egg yolks. Mix in chocolate chips, coconut, and walnuts. Mix well until fully combined.

3. Form cookies out of the mixture, and place them in the baking tray. Bake for 15 minutes until golden.

Nutritional Values per Serving:

Calories: **130** | Fat: **11.5**g | Protein: **2.9**g | Total Carbohydrates: **6**g | Dietary Fiber: **2.2**g | Net Carbohydrates: **3.8**g

9-Carrot Compact Cake

Diet Specs: GF | VEG

Yield: 16-cake balls/8-servings

Serving Portion: 2-cake balls

Preparation Time: 20 minutes

Cooking Time: 0 minutes

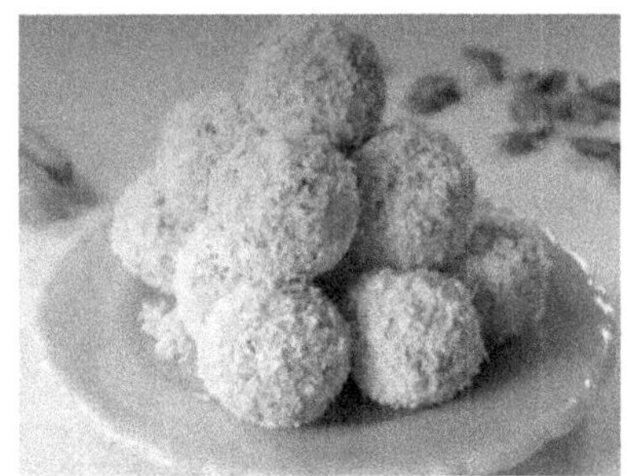

Ingredients:

1-block (8-oz.) cream cheese, softened

¾-cup coconut flour

1-tsp sweetener

½-tsp pure vanilla extract

1-tsp cinnamon

¼-tsp ground nutmeg

½-cup pecans, chopped

1-cup carrots, grated

1-cup unsweetened coconut, shredded

Directions:

1. Combine the first six ingredients in a large mixing bowl. Mix well by using a hand mixer until fully combined. Fold in the pecans and carrots.

2. Form 16 balls from the mixture, and roll each ball in shredded coconut.

Nutritional Values per Serving:

Calories: **94** | Fat: **8.3**g | Protein: **2.8**g | Total Carbohydrates: **5.2**g | Dietary Fiber: **3.1**g | Net Carbohydrates: **2.1**g

10-Chilled Cream

Diet Specs: GF | VEG | NF

Yield: 16-scoops/8-servings

Serving Portion: 2-ice cream scoops

Preparation Time: 8 hours 15 minutes

Cooking Time: 0 minutes

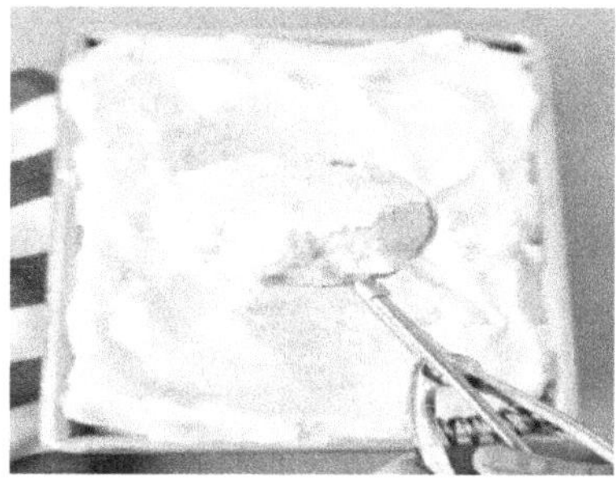

Ingredients:

2-cans (15-oz.) coconut milk, refrigerated for at least 3 hours

2-cups heavy cream

1-tsp pure vanilla extract

¼-cup sweetener

A pinch of kosher salt

Directions:

1. Spoon the refrigerated coconut milk into a large bowl. Leave the liquid in the can. By using a hand mixer, beat the milk until turning creamy. Set aside.

2. Beat the heavy cream in a separate large bowl until it forms soft peaks. Add the vanilla and sweetener. Beat again until fully combined.

3. Fold in the whipped milk into the whipped cream. Mix well and transfer the mixture in a loaf pan.

4. Place the pan in the freezer for 5 hours until the mixture becomes solid.

Nutritional Values per Serving:

Calories: **340** | Fat: **34.8**g | Protein: **3.7**g | Total Carbohydrates: **5.2**g | Dietary Fiber: **2.1**g | Net Carbohydrates: **3.1**g

Cooking Calibrations & Conversion Charts

For their popularity, all these ketogenic food recipes have found their way in a globally huge scale. This implies that they include several international versions with varying cooking measurements.

However, to facilitate your food shopping and cooking experiences, this book streamlines the cooking measurements of the recipes into the U.S. Customary Measurement Units. For further reference and convenience, the following charts present the most commonly used cooking measurements with their equivalents:

For measuring dry ingredients, measure them in graduated spoons and cups.

COMMON US DRY VOLUME MEASUREMENTS	
MEASURE	**EQUIVALENT**
a pinch	1/8-teaspoon
a dash	1/4-teaspoon
3-teaspoons	1-Tablespoon
1/8-cup	2-Tablespoons
1/4-cup	4-Tablespoons
1/3-cup	5-Tablespoons plus 1-teaspoon
1/2-cup	8-Tablespoons
3/4-cup	12-Tablespoons
1-cup	16-Tablespoons
1-pound	16-ounces

Except with those most critical cooking procedures and preparations, the British or Imperial measurements have the slightest variations with the International or Metric System compared to U.S. units. Thus, both the Metric and Imperial Systems are relatively the same.

For measuring liquid ingredients, the customary U.S. fluid ounce and British pint differ notably. To distinguish each, take note of their conversion factors:

◊ Convert U.S. pints into British pints by multiplying **0.83.**

◊ Convert U.S. fluid ounces into British fluid ounces by multiplying **1.04.**

COMMON US LIQUID VOLUME MEASUREMENTS	
MEASURE	**EQUIVALENT**
1-ounce	28-grams
8-fluid ounces	1-cup
1-pint	2-cups
1-quart	2-pints
1-gallon	4-quarts
1-teaspoon	5-ml
1-tablespoon	15-ml
1-cup	240-ml

Additionally, here are cooking temperature charts that explain at which oven or gas temperature range is ideal for your cooking applications:

OVEN TEMPERATURE RANGE, °F	COOKING APPLICATIONS
325 – 350 normal heat range	slow cooking/braising/cake baking to ensure a Maillard reaction or the browning of proteins, as well as caramelization or the browning of sugars
375 – 400 medium-high heat	shorter term roasting/baking to ensure desirable appearances of bubbling golden cheese, crisp edges to cookies, and crisp golden skin to chicken
425 – 450 high heat	short-term roasting/baking to ensure pastries with a golden color puff
475 – 500 ultra-high heat	baking breads/pizza shells since it allows the dough to rise before the gluten has any chances to set

OVEN TEMPERATURE CONVERSION CHART		
Fahrenheit, °F	**Celsius, °C**	**Gas Mark Rating**
275	140	1-cool
300	150	2
325	165	3-very moderate
350	180	4-moderate
375	190	5
400	200	6-moderately hot
425	220	7- hot
450	230	9
475	240	10- very hot

To guide further you with other important cooking measurement conversions, check your preferences with this summarized chart:

US TO METRIC CONVERSIONS	
1/5-teaspoon	1-mL
1-teaspoon	5-ml
1-tablespoon	15-ml
1-fluid ounce	30-ml
3.4-fluid ounce	100-ml
34-fluid ounce	1-liter
1/5-cup	50-ml
1-cup	240-ml
2-cups (1-pint)	470-ml
2.1-pints	1-liter
4-cups (1-quart)	0.95-liter
4.2-cups	1-liter
1.06-quarts	1-liter
4-quarts (1-gallon)	3.8-liters
0.26-gallon	1-liter
0.035-ounce	1-gram
1-oz.	28-grams
3.5-oz.	100-grams
35-oz.	1-kilogram
1-pound	454-grams
1.10-pounds	500-grams
2.205-pounds	1-kilogram

Chapter 10-Daily Dietary Planning Programs

Plan and organize your diet; diet on your organized plan! Start to plan for seven days' worth of your ketogenic diet recipes, and you will save much of your precious time, effort, and money in the process.

Bear in mind, it would be a whole lot easier going to a restaurant or cooking an instant convenience food when everybody at home is hungry or you still have to prepare or defrost food stocks; nonetheless, a little planning will let you go a long, long way to avoid such diversions from your diet!

Your 7-day meal plan will be guiding you to program the entire duration of your scheduled daily meals while making your food shopping and cooking experiences easier than ever. All the recipes that compose your meal plan will be the recipes presented in this book.

Hence, squeeze your creative juices and explore mixing and matching up your daily cooking routines with your recipes. You should be able to look and shop for all the ingredients of the recipes since they are easily available and accessible in most supermarkets, wherever your location is. In the end, your ketogenic diet meal-planning program will be your essential tool for maintaining and sustaining your dietary change in accordance with your intended calorie consumption!

Calorie Consumption Calculation

For fitness buffs, especially when you are focusing more about total wellness with your ketogenic dietary journey, you should be aware of your *recommended daily calorie intake* (RDCI) value. You can actually calculate manually your estimated RDCI value.

You should first understand your *Basal Metabolic Rate* (BMR). The BMR is essentially the number of calories you would have been burning if you were in bed all day or not in any way performing a moderate or strenuous physical activity. However, this rate differs in gender. Initially, you calculate for your BMR by using the following formula:

INDIVIDUAL	BASAL METABOLIC RATE (BMR) FORMULA
MEN	66 + (13.7 x WEIGHT IN KILOGRAMS) + (5 x HEIGHT IN CM) − (6.8 x AGE IN YEARS)
WOMEN	65 + (9.6 x WEIGHT IN KILOGRAMS) + (1.8 x HEIGHT IN CM) − (4.7 x AGE IN YEARS)

Subsequently, you calculate for the proximate value of your RDCI by using the *Harris-Benedict Formula* (as demonstrated on the following chart). The formula actually factors the various intensity levels of your day-to-day physical activities such as your daily physical fitness training, work, and routines with respect to your calculated BMR:

DAILY ACTIVITY INTENSITY LEVEL	HARRIS-BENEDICT FORMULA
Least Active little or no exercise	BMR x 1.2
Lightly Active light exercise/work 1-3 days per week	BMR x 1.375
Moderately Active moderate exercise/work 3-5 days per week	BMR x 1.55
Very Active hard exercise/work 6-7 days a week	BMR x 1.725
Extra Active very hard exercise/work 6-7 days a week	BMR x 1.9

The following daily meal plans derive RDCI values of [1,500], [1,750], and [2,000], which will be dependent on your corresponding BMR results to help you to either maintain or reduce your weight. Your RDCI indicates how much macronutrients contained in a serving portion of food that will contribute to your daily ketogenic diet.

7-Day Dietary Planning Program (1,500 Calorie Consumption)

Starting and sticking to a daily 1,500-calorie meal plan can be challenging; however, if you only know your daily allowances for each food group or macronutrient consumption, then it can help you to know what to eat and plan a dietary program that is both nutritious and fulfilling.

To be more precise on reducing calorie intakes to help you shed off healthy pounds per week, calculate your daily calorie goal by multiplying your present weight by 12. The result denotes your basic daily calorie consumption. If your goal is to:

- Lose 1 pound per week, cut down 500 calories a day

- Lose 2 pounds per week, cut down 1,000 calories a day

Hence, if you are currently weighing 150 pounds and you aim is to lose one pound weekly, then:

150 [pounds] x 12 = 1,800 [calories]

1,800 [calories] − 500 [calories] = 1,300 calories

However, this formula assumes that you are sedentary. Otherwise, you need to take more calories than you initially calculated to feel full during the day. Your ideal gauge for whether you are indeed losing weight or at the proper level of cutting down your calories will be how satisfied you feel. You should never be hungry all day!

If you are still unsure, begin safely with a 1,500-calorie ketogenic diet plan. For, after all, this level is where most people are able to lose weight. You can eat delicious foods, albeit, low in calories while feeling full when following this easy diet meal plan:

DAY-1	KETOGENIC MEALS	SERVING PORTION	NUTRITIONAL VALUES PER SERVING	
BREAKFAST	Spinach Sausage Feta Frittata	1-frittata wedge	Calories: **295** | Fat: **22.9g** | Protein: **18.5g** | Total Carbs: **4.6g** | Dietary Fiber: **1g** | Net Carbs: **3.6g**	
SNACK	Choco Coco Cups	2-mini cups	Calories: **240** | Fat: **25.3g** | Protein: **2.1g** | Total Carbs: **5g** | Dietary Fiber: **4g** | Net Carbs: **1g**	
LUNCH	Smoky Sage Sausage	1-patty	Calories: **170** | Fat: **13.2g** | Protein: **8.4g** | Total Carbs: **5.3g** | Dietary Fiber: **1g** | Net Carbs: **4.3g**	
LUNCH	Coco Crack Bake-less Biscuit Bars	1-biscuit bar	Calories: **106** | Fat: **10.5g** | Protein: **3g** | Total Carbs: **2.3g** | Dietary Fiber: **2g** | Net Carbs: **0.3g**	
SNACK	Ambrosial Avocado Puree Pudding	1-glass	Calories: **240** | Fat: **23.8g** | Protein: **2.8g** | Total Carbs: **12.8g** | Dietary Fiber: **9g** | Net Carbs: **3.8g**	
DINNER	Grain-less Gnocchi in Melted Mozzarella	1-serving bowl	Calories: **355** | Fat: **27.6g** | Protein: **22.1g** | Total Carbs: **6.5g** | Dietary Fiber: **2.1g** | Net Carbs: **4.4g**	
DINNER	Carrot Compact Cake	2-cake balls	Calories: **94** | Fat: **8.3g** | Protein: **2.8g** | Total Carbs: **5.2g** | Dietary Fiber: **3.1g** | Net Carbs: **2.1g**	
TOTAL CALORIE CONSUMPTION			1,500	
FAT			131.6g	78.9%
PROTEIN			59.7g	15.9%
NET CARBOHYDRATES			19.5g	5.2%

DAY-2	KETOGENIC MEALS	SERVING PORTION	NUTRITIONAL VALUES PER SERVING	
BREAKFAST	Hearty Hodgepodge	1-serving bowl	Calories: **290** | Fat: **24**g | Protein: **14.6** g | Total Carbs: **6.7**g | Dietary Fiber: **3.1**g | Net Carbs: **3.6**g	
SNACK	Coconut Candy	4-candy balls	Calories: **204** | Fat: **17.2**g | Protein: **10.2**g | Total Carbs: **3**g | Dietary Fiber: **0.8**g | Net Carbs: **2.2**g	
LUNCH	Pulled Pepper-Lemon Loins	1-chicken loin	Calories: **280** | Fat: **23.3**g | Protein: **14**g | Total Carbs: **4.1**g | Dietary Fiber: **0.6**g | Net Carbs: **3.5**g	
	Butter Ball Bombs	3-butter balls	Calories: **51** | Fat: **4.3**g | Protein: **0.7**g | Total Carbs: **2.7**g | Dietary Fiber: **0.4**g | Net Carbs: **2.3**g	
SNACK	Philadelphia Potato Praline	4-pralines	Calories: **180** | Fat: **15.3**g | Protein: **8.9**g | Total Carbs: **3.2**g | Dietary Fiber: **1.5**g | Net Carbs: **1.7**g	
DINNER	Soba & Spinach Sprouts	1-serving bowl	Calories: **355** | Fat: **29.6**g | Protein: **17.8**g | Total Carbs: **8.3**g | Dietary Fiber: **3.9**g | Net Carbs: **4.4**g	
	Matcha Muffins with Choco-Coco Coating	2-muffins	Calories: **140** | Fat: **10.9**g | Protein: **5.1**g | Total Carbs: **8.8**g | Dietary Fiber: **3.4**g | Net Carbs: **5.4**g	
TOTAL CALORIE CONSUMPTION			1,500	
FAT			124.6g	74.8%
PROTEIN			71.3g	19.0%
NET CARBOHYDRATES			23.1g	6.2%

DAY-3	KETOGENIC MEALS	SERVING PORTION	NUTRITIONAL VALUES PER SERVING	
BREAKFAST	Avocado Aliment with Egg Element	1-halved stuffed avocado	Calories: **275** | Fat: **23.8g** | Protein: **11.8g** | Total Carbs: **7.4g** | Dietary Fiber: **4g** | Net Carbs: **3.4g**	
SNACK	Power-Packed Butter Balls	2-balls	Calories: **128** | Fat: **10.1g** | Protein: **4.9g** | Total Carbs: **7.2g** | Dietary Fiber: **2.9g** | Net Carbs: **4.3g**	
LUNCH	Aubergine Á la Lasagna Lunch	1-lasagna slice	Calories: **346** | Fat: **27g** | Protein: **21.4g** | Total Carbs: **7.9g** | Dietary Fiber: **3.5g** | Net Carbs: **4.4g**	
	Chocolate-Coated Sweet Strawberries	2-candy cubes	Calories: **125** | Fat: **11.1g** | Protein: **2.7g** | Total Carbs: **5g** | Dietary Fiber: **1.4g** | Net Carbs: **3.6g**	
SNACK	Corndog Clumps	2-corndogs	Calories: **148** | Fat: **13.2g** | Protein: **3.9g** | Total Carbs: **4g** | Dietary Fiber: **1.6g** | Net Carbs: **3.4g**	
DINNER	Cheesy Cauliflower Mac Munchies	1-serving bowl	Calories: **352** | Fat: **27.8g** | Protein: **20.9g** | Total Carbs: **8.9g** | Dietary Fiber: **4.3g** | Net Carbs: **4.6g**	
	Choco Coco Cookies	3-cookies	Calories: **130** | Fat: **11.5g** | Protein: **2.9g** | Total Carbs: **6g** | Dietary Fiber: **2.2g** | Net Carbos: **3.8g**	
TOTAL CALORIE CONSUMPTION			1,504	
FAT			124.5g	74.5%
PROTEIN			68.5g	18.2%
NET CARBOHYDRATES			27.5g	7.3%

DAY-4	KETOGENIC MEALS	SERVING PORTION	NUTRITIONAL VALUES PER SERVING	
BREAKFAST	Avocados atop Toasted Tartiné	1-tartiné	Calories: 268	Fat: 22.4g	Protein: 13.5g	Total Carbs: 8.9g	Dietary Fiber: 6.7g	Net Carbs: 3.2g	
SNACK	Tasty Turkey Cheese Cylinders	2-rollups	Calories: 162	Fat: 10.9g	Protein: 15.6g	Total Carbs: 3.8g	Dietary Fiber: 0g	Net Carbs: 3.8g	
LUNCH	Sautéed Sirloin Steak in Sour Sauce	1-serving bowl	Calories: 350	Fat: 29.3g	Protein: 17.7g	Total Carbs: 4.9g	Dietary Fiber: 1g	Net Carbs: 3.9g	
	Carrot Compact Cake	2-cake balls	Calories: 94	Fat: 8.3g	Protein: 2.8g	Total Carbs: 5.2g	Dietary Fiber: 3.1g	Net Carbs: 2.1g	
SNACK	Fried Flaxseed Tortilla Treat	2-shells flaxseed tortillas	Calories: 36	Fat: 2.8g	Protein: 0.8g	Total Carbs: 2.7g	Dietary Fiber: 0.7g	Net Carbs: 2g	
DINNER	Chicken Cauliflower Curry	1-serving bowl	Calories: 334	Fat: 27g	Protein: 18.7g	Total Carbs: 8.4g	Dietary Fiber: 4.3g	Net Carbs: 4.1g	
	Cinnamon Cup Cake	1-cup cake	Calories: 263	Fat: 24.1g	Protein: 7.6g	Total Carbs: 14.2g	Dietary Fiber: 10.3g	Net Carbs: 3.9g	
TOTAL CALORIE CONSUMPTION			1,507	
FAT			124.8g	74.5%
PROTEIN			76.7g	20.4%
NET CARBOHYDRATES			23.0g	6.1%

DAY-5	KETOGENIC MEALS	SERVING PORTION	NUTRITIONAL VALUES PER SERVING	
BREAKFAST	Seasoned Sardines with Sunny Side	1-serving bowl	Calories: **255** | Fat: **21g** | Protein: **13.5g** | Total Carbs: **4.9g** | Dietary Fiber: **1.8g** | Net Carbs: **3.1g**	
SNACK	Mozzarella Mound Munchies	1-cheese mound	Calories: **157** | Fat: **13.2g** | Protein: **5.9g** | Total Carbs: **4.8g** | Dietary Fiber: **1.1g** | Net Carbs: **3.7g**	
LUNCH	Beef Broccoli with Sesame Sauce	1-serving bowl	Calories: **375** | Fat: **31g** | Protein: **19.5g** | Total Carbs: **5.4g** | Dietary Fiber: **0.8g** | Net Carbs: **4.6g**	
	Cinnamon Cup Cake	1-cup cake	Calories: **263** | Fat: **24.1g** | Protein: **7.6g** | Total Carbs: **14.2g** | Dietary Fiber: **10.3g** | Net Carbs: **3.9g**	
SNACK	Kingly Kale Crispy Chips	1-serving bowl	Calories: **81** | Fat: **7.6g** | Protein: **1.9g** | Total Carbs: **2.1g** | Dietary Fiber: **0.9g** | Net Carbs: **1.2g**	
DINNER	Zesty Zucchini Pseudo Pasta & Sweet Spanish Onions Overload	1-serving bowl	Calories: **319** | Fat: **25.9g** | Protein: **18.1g** | Total Carbs: **6.6g** | Dietary Fiber: **3.2g** | Net Carbs: **3.4g**	
	Butter Ball Bombs	3-butter balls	Calories: **51** | Fat: **4.3g** | Protein: **0.7g** | Total Carbs: **2.7g** | Dietary Fiber: **0.4g** | Net Carbs: **2.3g**	
TOTAL CALORIE CONSUMPTION			1,501	
FAT			127.1g	76.2%
PROTEIN			67.2g	17.9%
NET CARBOHYDRATES			22.2g	5.9%

DAY-6	KETOGENIC MEALS	SERVING PORTION	NUTRITIONAL VALUES PER SERVING	
BREAKFAST	Blueberries Breakfast Bowl	1-serving bowl	Calories: **202** | Fat: **16.8g** | Protein: **10.2g** | Total Carbs: **9.8g** | Dietary Fiber: **5.8g** | Net Carbs: **2.6g**	
SNACK	Ambrosial Avocado Puree Pudding	1-glass	Calories: **240** | Fat: **23.8g** | Protein: **2.8g** | Total Carbs: **12.8g** | Dietary Fiber: **9g** | Net Carbs: **3.8g**	
LUNCH	Chicken Curry Masala Mix	1-serving bowl	Calories: **377** | Fat: **29.3g** | Protein: **23.4g** | Total Carbs: **6.8g** | Dietary Fiber: **1.9g** | Net Carbos: **4.9g**	
LUNCH	Butter Ball Bombs	3-butter balls	Calories: **51** | Fat: **4.3g** | Protein: **0.7g** | Total Carbs: **2.7g** | Dietary Fiber: **0.4g** | Net Carbs: **2.3g**	
SNACK	Choco Coco Cups	2-mini cups	Calories: **240** | Fat: **25.3g** | Protein: **2.1g** | Total Carbs: **5g** | Dietary Fiber: **4g** | Net Carbs: **1g**	
DINNER	All-Avocado Stuffed with Spicy Beef Bits	1-halved stuffed avocado	Calories: **280** | Fat: **23.1g** | Protein: **14g** | Total Carbs: **6.3g** | Dietary Fiber: **2.2g** | Net Carbs: **4.1g**	
DINNER	Cool Cucumber Sushi with Sriracha Sauce	3-sushi slices	Calories: **110** | Fat: **10.1g** | Protein: **1.9g** | Total Carbs: **4.8g** | Dietary Fiber: **2g** | Net Carbs: **2.8g**	
TOTAL CALORIE CONSUMPTION			1,500	
FAT			132.7g	79.6%
PROTEIN			55.1g	14.7%
NET CARBOHYDRATES			21.5g	5.7%

DAY-7	KETOGENIC MEALS	SERVING PORTION	NUTRITIONAL VALUES PER SERVING	
BREAKFAST	Pumpkin Pancakes	2-pancakes	Calories: **200** | Fat: **16.4**g | Protein: **11**g | Total Carbs: **5.2**g | Dietary Fiber: **3**g | Net Carbs: **2.2**g	
SNACK	Fried Flaxseed Tortilla Treat	2-shells flaxseed tortillas	Calories: **36** | Fat: **2.8**g | Protein: **0.8**g | Total Carbs: **2.7**g | Dietary Fiber: **0.7**g | Net Carbs: **2**g	
LUNCH	Chickpeas Carrots Curry	1-serving bowl	Calories: **380** | Fat: **30.9**g | Protein: **18**g | Total Carbs: **14.4**g | Dietary Fiber: **10.7**g | Net Carbs: **3.7**g	
	Matcha Muffins with Choco-Coco Coating	2-muffins	Calories: **140** | Fat: **10.9**g | Protein: **5.1**g | Total Carbs: **8.8**g | Dietary Fiber: **3.4**g | Net Carbs: **5.4**g	
SNACK	Tasty Turkey Cheese Cylinders	2-rollups	Calories: **162** | Fat: **10.9**g | Protein: **15.6**g | Total Carbs: **3.8**g | Dietary Fiber: **0**g | Net Carbs: **3.8**g	
DINNER	Spicy & Smoky Spinach-Set Fish Fillets	1-fish fillet	Calories: **248** | Fat: **18.8**g | Protein: **15.3**g | Total Carbs: **13.2**g | Dietary Fiber: **8.9**g | Net Carbs: **4.3**g	
	Chilled Cream	2-ice cream scoops	Calories: **340** | Fat: **34.8**g | Protein: **3.7**g | Total Carbs: **5.2**g | Dietary Fiber: **2.1**g | Net Carbs: **3.1**g	
TOTAL CALORIE CONSUMPTION			1,506	
FAT			125.5g	75.0%
PROTEIN			69.5g	18.5%
NET CARBOHYDRATES			24.5g	6.5%

7-Day Dietary Planning Program (1,750 Calorie Consumption)

Calorie consumption really depends on the number of calories you expend per day with your routine activities. Again, you actually base it on your weight goals.

Hence, when you are eating 1,750 calories a day, yet, only expend 1500, you will certainly gain weight. Conversely, when you are eating 1,750 calories a day, yet, expend 1900, you will definitely lose weight. As always, define your plans and keep a balance in accordance with your intents.

DAY-1	KETOGENIC MEALS	SERVING PORTION	NUTRITIONAL VALUES PER SERVING
BREAKFAST	Cream Cheese Protein Pancake	2-pancakes	Calories: 340 | Fat: 28.6g | Protein: 16.2g | Total Carbs: 8.1g | Dietary Fiber: 3.8g | Net Carbs: 4.3g
SNACKS	Choco Coco Cups	2-mini cups	Calories: 240 | Fat: 25.3g | Protein: 2.1g | Total Carbs: 5g | Dietary Fiber: 4g | Net Carbs: 1g
LUNCH	Crispy Chicken Packed in Pandan	1-chicken thigh	Calories: 382 | Fat: 32.5g | Protein: 17.8g | Total Carbs: 7.7g | Dietary Fiber: 3.1g | Net Carbs: 4.6g
	Choco 'Cado Twin Truffles	3-candy balls	Calories: 68 | Fat: 5.8g | Protein: 1.6g | Total Carbs: 4.2g | Dietary Fiber: 1.8g | Net Carbs: 2.4g
SNACKS	Philadelphia Potato Praline	4-pralines	Calories: 180 | Fat: 15.3g | Protein: 8.9g | Total Carbs: 3.2g | Dietary Fiber: 1.5g | Net Carbs: 1.7g
DINNER	Therapeutic Turmeric & Shirataki Soup	1-serving bowl	Calories: 415 | Fat: 34.6g | Protein: 21.6g | Total Carbs: 10.1g | Dietary Fiber: 5.7g | Net Carbs: 4.4g
	Chocolate-Coated Sweet Strawberries	2-candy cubes	Calories: 125 | Fat: 11.1g | Protein: 2.7g | Total Carbs: 5g | Dietary Fiber: 1.4g | Net Carbs: 3.6g
TOTAL CALORIE CONSUMPTION			1,750
FAT			153.2g | 78.8%
PROTEIN			70.9g | 16.2%
NET CARBOHYDRATES			22.0g | 5.0%

DAY-2	KETOGENIC MEALS	SERVING PORTION	NUTRITIONAL VALUES PER SERVING	
BREAKFAST	Feta-Filled Tomato-Topped Oldie Omelet	1-omelet	Calories: **335** | Fat: **28.4**g | Protein: **16.2**g | Total Carbs: **4.5**g | Dietary Fiber: **0.8**g | Net Carbs: **3.7**g	
SNACKS	Ambrosial Avocado Puree Pudding	1-glass	Calories: **240** | Fat: **23.8**g | Protein: **2.8**g | Total Carbs: **12.8**g | Dietary Fiber: **9**g | Net Carbs: **3.8**g	
LUNCH	Tasty Tofu Carrots &Cauliflower Cereal	1-serving bowl	Calories: **390** | Fat: **32.6**g | Protein: **19.5**g | Total Carbs: **17.4**g | Dietary Fiber: **12.7**g | Net Carbs: **4.7**g	
	Coco Crack Bake-less Bounty Bars	1-bar	Calories: **106** | Fat: **10.5**g | Protein: **2.9**g | Total Carbs: **2**g | Dietary Fiber: **2**g | Net Carbs: **0**g	
SNACKS	Mozzarella Mound Munchies	1-cheese mound	Calories: **157** | Fat: **13.2**g | Protein: **5.9**g | Total Carbs: **4.8**g | Dietary Fiber: **1.1**g | Net Carbs: **3.7**g	
DINNER	À la Spaghetti with Asian Sauce	1-serving plate	Calories: **412** | Fat: **34.4**g | Protein: **20.9**g | Total Carbs: **10.5**g | Dietary Fiber: **5.7**g | Net Carbs: **4.8**g	
	Cool Cucumber Sushi with Sriracha Sauce	3-sushi slices	Calories: **110** | Fat: **10.1**g | Protein: **1.9**g | Total Carbs: **4.8**g | Dietary Fiber: **2**g | Net Carbs: **2.8**g	
TOTAL CALORIE CONSUMPTION			1,750	
FAT			153.0g	78.6%
PROTEIN			70.1g	16.0%
NET CARBOHYDRATES			23.5g	5.4%

DAY-3	KETOGENIC MEALS	SERVING PORTION	NUTRITIONAL VALUES PER SERVING	
BREAKFAST	Whole-Wheat Plain Pancakes	2-pancakes	Calories: **329** | Fat: **27.6**g | Protein: **16.1**g | Total Carbs: **5.4**g | Dietary Fiber: **1.3**g | Net Carbs: **4.4**g	
SNACKS	Coconut Candy	4-candy balls	Calories: **204** | Fat: **17.2**g | Protein: **10.2**g | Total Carbs: **3**g | Dietary Fiber: **0.8**g | Net Carbs: **2.2**g	
LUNCH	Steamed Salmon & Salad Bento Box	1-bento box	Calories: **391** | Fat: **30.4**g | Protein: **24.9**g | Total Carbs: **11.8**g | Dietary Fiber: **7.3**g | Net Carbs: **4.5**g	
	Chocolate-Coated Sweet Strawberries	2-candy cubes	Calories: **125** | Fat: **11.1**g | Protein: **2.7**g | Total Carbs: **5**g | Dietary Fiber: **1.4**g | Net Carbs: **3.6**g	
SNACKS	Fried Flaxseed Tortilla Treat	2-shells flaxseed tortillas	Calories: **36** | Fat: **2.8**g | Protein: **0.8**g | Total Carbs: **2.7**g | Dietary Fiber: **0.7**g | Net Carbs: **2**g	
DINNER	Cheddar Chicken Casserole	1-serving plate	Calories: **405** | Fat: **33.8**g | Protein: **22.7**g | Total Carbs: **3.6**g | Dietary Fiber: **1**g | Net Carbs: **2.6**g	
	Cinnamon Cup Cake	1-cup cake	Calories: **263** | Fat: **24.1**g | Protein: **7.6**g | Total Carbs: **14.2**g | Dietary Fiber: **10.3**g | Net Carbs: **3.9**g	
TOTAL CALORIE CONSUMPTION			1,753	
FAT			147.0g	75.4%
PROTEIN			85.0g	19.3%
NET CARBOHYDRATES			23.2g	5.3%

DAY-4	KETOGENIC MEALS	SERVING PORTION	NUTRITIONAL VALUES PER SERVING	
BREAKFAST	Romantic Raspberry Power Pancake	2-pancakes	Calories: **323** | Fat: **25.3**g | Protein: **15.7**g | Total Carbs: **12**g | Dietary Fiber: **3.8**g | Net Carbs: **4.8**g	
SNACKS	Tasty Turkey Cheese Cylinders	2-rollups	Calories: **162** | Fat: **10.9**g | Protein: **15.6**g | Total Carbs: **3.8**g | Dietary Fiber: **0**g | Net Carbs: **3.8**g	
LUNCH	Prawn Pasta	1-serving plate	Calories: **393** | Fat: **32.8**g | Protein: **19.7**g | Total Carbs: **14.9**g | Dietary Fiber: **10.1**g | Net Carbs: **4.8**g	
	Chilled Cream	2-ice cream scoops	Calories: **340** | Fat: **34.8**g | Protein: **3.7**g | Total Carbs: **5.2**g | Dietary Fiber: **2.1**g | Net Carbs: **3.1**g	
SNACKS	Kingly Kale Crispy Chips	1-serving bowl	Calories: **81** | Fat: **7.6**g | Protein: **1.9**g | Total Carbs: **2.1**g | Dietary Fiber: **0.9**g | Net Carbs: **1.2**g	
DINNER	Sugar Snap Pea Pods with Coco Crunch	1-serving bowl	Calories: **389** | Fat: **31.3**g | Protein: **22**g | Total Carbs: **7.2**g | Dietary Fiber: **2.3**g | Net Carbs: **4.9**g	
	Choco 'Cado Twin Truffles	3-candy balls	Calories: **68** | Fat: **5.8**g | Protein: **1.6**g | Total Carbs: **4.2**g | Dietary Fiber: **1.8**g | Net Carbs: **2.4**g	
TOTAL CALORIE CONSUMPTION			1,756	
FAT			148.5g	76.1%
PROTEIN			80.2g	18.2%
NET CARBOHYDRATES			25.0g	5.7%

DAY-5	KETOGENIC MEALS	SERVING PORTION	NUTRITIONAL VALUES PER SERVING	
BREAKFAST	Spinach Shoots Mediterranean Medley	1-serving bowl	Calories: **308**	Fat: **26**g	Protein: **15.4**g	Total Carbs: **9.7**g	Dietary Fiber: **6.5**g	Net Carbs: **3.2**g	
SNACKS	Choco Coco Cups	2-mini cups	Calories: **240**	Fat: **25.3**g	Protein: **2.1**g	Total Carbs: **5**g	Dietary Fiber: **4**g	Net Carbs: **1**g	
LUNCH	Flaky Fillets with Garden Greens	1-fish fillet	Calories: **395**	Fat: **33**g	Protein: **19.8**g	Total Carbs: **8.7**g	Dietary Fiber: **3.9**g	Net Carbs: **4.8**g	
LUNCH	Matcha Muffins with Choco-Coco Coating	2-muffins	Calories: **140**	Fat: **10.9**g	Protein: **5.1**g	Total Carbs: **8.8**g	Dietary Fiber: **3.4**g	Net Carbs: **5.4**g	
SNACKS	Mozzarella Mound Munchies	1-cheese mound	Calories: **157**	Fat: **13.2**g	Protein: **5.9**g	Total Carbs: **4.8**g	Dietary Fiber: **1.1**g	Net Carbs: **3.7**g	
DINNER	Pizza Pie with Cheesy Cauliflower Crust	2-pizza wedges	Calories: **384**	Fat: **32.1**g	Protein: **19.9**g	Total Carbs: **5.5**g	Dietary Fiber: **1.7**g	Net Carbs: **3.8**g	
DINNER	Choco Coco Cookies	3-cookies	Calories: **130**	Fat: **11.5**g	Protein: **2.9**g	Total Carbs: **6**g	Dietary Fiber: **2.2**g	Net Carbos: **3.8**g	
TOTAL CALORIE CONSUMPTION			1,754	
FAT			152.0 g	78.0%
PROTEIN			71.1 g	16.2%
NET CARBOHYDRATES			25.7 g	5.8%

DAY-6	KETOGENIC MEALS	SERVING PORTION	NUTRITIONAL VALUES PER SERVING
BREAKFAST	Fish Fillet & Perky Potato Cheese Combo	1-serving plate	Calories: **298** | Fat: **24.9g** | Protein: **14.2g** | Total Carbs: **6.5g** | Dietary Fiber: **3.2g** | Net Carbs: **4.3g**
SNACKS	Kingly Kale Crispy Chips	1-serving bowl	Calories: **81** | Fat: **7.6g** | Protein: **1.9g** | Total Carbs: **2.1g** | Dietary Fiber: **0.9g** | Net Carbs: **1.2g**
LUNCH	Milano Meatballs with Tangy Tomato	2-meatballs	Calories: **396** | Fat: **32.6g** | Protein: **20.9g** | Total Carbs: **8.2g** | Dietary Fiber: **3.4g** | Net Carbs: **4.8g**
	Choco Coco Cookies	3-cookies	Calories: **130** | Fat: **11.5g** | Protein: **2.9g** | Total Carbs: **6g** | Dietary Fiber: **2.2g** | Net Carbos: **3.8g**
SNACKS	Power-Packed Butter Balls	2-balls	Calories: **128** | Fat: **10.1g** | Protein: **4.9g** | Total Carbs: **7.2g** | Dietary Fiber: **2.9g** | Net Carbs: **4.3g**
DINNER	Spaghetti-Styled Zesty Zucchini with Guacamole Garnish	1-set guacamole and carbonara	Calories: **381** | Fat: **31.8g** | Protein: **19g** | Total Carbs: **14.3g** | Dietary Fiber: **9.5g** | Net Carbs: **4.8g**
	Chilled Cream	2-ice cream scoops	Calories: **340** | Fat: **34.8g** | Protein: **3.7g** | Total Carbs: **5.2g** | Dietary Fiber: **2.1g** | Net Carbs: **3.1g**
TOTAL CALORIE CONSUMPTION			1,754
FAT			153.3g / 78.6%
PROTEIN			67.5g / 15.4%
NET CARBOHYDRATES			26.3g / 6.0%

DAY-7	KETOGENIC MEALS	SERVING PORTION	NUTRITIONAL VALUES PER SERVING
BREAKFAST	Mayonnaise Mixed with Energy Egg	1-serving bowl	Calories: 295 | Fat: 22.7g | Protein: 18.8g | Total Carbs: 3.8g | Dietary Fiber: 0.1g | Net Carbs: 3.7g
SNACKS	Choco Coco Cups	2-mini cups	Calories: 240 | Fat: 25.3g | Protein: 2.1g | Total Carbs: 5g | Dietary Fiber: 4g | Net Carbs: 1g
LUNCH	Stuffed Straw Mushroom Mobcap	1-cup stuffed mushroom	Calories: 401 | Fat: 34.7g | Protein: 17.2g | Total Carbs: 16.9g | Dietary Fiber: 11.4g | Net Carbs: 5g
LUNCH	Cool Cucumber Sushi with Sriracha Sauce	3-sushi slices	Calories: 110 | Fat: 10.1g | Protein: 1.9g | Total Carbs: 4.8g | Dietary Fiber: 2g | Net Carbs: 2.8g
SNACKS	Ambrosial Avocado Puree Pudding	1-glass	Calories: 240 | Fat: 23.8g | Protein: 2.8g | Total Carbs: 12.8g | Dietary Fiber: 9g | Net Carbs: 3.8g
DINNER	Spicy Shrimps & Sweet Shishito	1-serving bowl	Calories: 370 | Fat: 28.9g | Protein: 23g | Total Carbs: 7.2g | Dietary Fiber: 2.8g | Net Carbs: 4.4g
DINNER	Carrot Compact Cake	2-cake balls	Calories: 94 | Fat: 8.3g | Protein: 2.8g | Total Carbs: 5.2g | Dietary Fiber: 3.1g | Net Carbs: 2.1g
TOTAL CALORIE CONSUMPTION			1,750
FAT			153.8g — 79.1%
PROTEIN			68.6g — 15.7%
NET CARBOHYDRATES			22.8g — 5.2%

7- Day Dietary Planning Program (2,000 Calorie Consumption)

For all intents of providing the most helpful nutritional information to consumers, the Food and Drug Administration (FDA) of the U.S. uses a 2,000-calorie regimen as the standard model for the entire *Nutrition Facts* label on foods. The label generally provides information about *Percentage Daily Value* (%-DV).

However, the model is not a recommendation that you ought to consume 2,000 calories a day. Moreover, it does not indicate that a 2,000-calorie regimen is worse or necessarily better than, say, a 2,500-calorie or a 1,200-calorie diet. As your constant reminder, if you were trying to gain or lose weight with the facilitation of the ketogenic diet, then you would simply adjust your daily caloric intake to reach your specific health goals.

DAY-**1**	KETOGENIC MEALS	SERVING PORTION	NUTRITIONAL VALUES PER SERVING	
BREAKFAST	Choco Chip Whey Waffles	2-waffles	Calories: **423** | Fat: **32.8g** | Protein: **26.5g** | Total Carbs: **8.3g** | Dietary Fiber: **2.9g** | Net Carbs: **5.4g**	
SNACKS	Ambrosial Avocado Puree Pudding	1-glass	Calories: **240** | Fat: **23.8g** | Protein: **2.8g** | Total Carbs: **12.8g** | Dietary Fiber: **9g** | Net Carbs: **3.8g**	
LUNCH	Stuffed Straw Mushroom Mobcap	1-cup stuffed mushroom	Calories: **401** | Fat: **34.7g** | Protein: **17.2g** | Total Carbs: **16.9g** | Dietary Fiber: **11.4g** | Net Carbs: **5g**	
	Coco Crack Bake-less Bounty Bars	1-bar	Calories: **106** | Fat: **10.5g** | Protein: **2.9g** | Total Carbs: **2g** | Dietary Fiber: **2g** | Net Carbs: **0g**	
SNACKS	Choco Coco Cups	2-mini cups	Calories: **240** | Fat: **25.3g** | Protein: **2.1g** | Total Carbs: **5g** | Dietary Fiber: **4g** | Net Carbs: **1g**	
DINNER	Cauliflower Chao Fan Fried with Pork Pastiche	1-serving bowl	Calories: **460** | Fat: **35.7g** | Protein: **28.6g** | Total Carbs: **8.3g** | Dietary Fiber: **2.3g** | Net Carbs: **6g**	
	Choco Coco Cookies	3-cookies	Calories: **130** | Fat: **11.5g** | Protein: **2.9g** | Total Carbs: **6g** | Dietary Fiber: **2.2g** | Net Carbos: **3.8g**	
TOTAL CALORIE CONSUMPTION			2,000	
FAT			174.3g	78.4%
PROTEIN			83.0g	16.6%
NET CARBOHYDRATES			25.0g	5.0%

DAY-2	KETOGENIC MEALS	SERVING PORTION	NUTRITIONAL VALUES PER SERVING	
BREAKFAST	Magdalena Muffins with Tart Tomatoes	2-muffins	Calories: **405** | Fat: **33.3g** | Protein: **20.3g** | Total Carbs: **11g** | Dietary Fiber: **4.9g** | Net Carbs: **6.1g**	
SNACKS	Corndog Clumps	2-corndogs	Calories: **148** | Fat: **13.2g** | Protein: **3.9g** | Total Carbs: **4g** | Dietary Fiber: **1.6g** | Net Carbs: **3.4g**	
LUNCH	Stuffed Spaghetti Squash	1-halved stuffed squash	Calories: **404** | Fat: **33.2g** | Protein: **20.3g** | Total Carbs: **7g** | Dietary Fiber: **1g** | Net Carbs: **6g**	
	Matcha Muffins with Choco-Coco Coating	2-muffins	Calories: **140** | Fat: **10.9g** | Protein: **5.1g** | Total Carbs: **8.8g** | Dietary Fiber: **3.4g** | Net Carbs: **5.4g**	
SNACKS	Philadelphia Potato Praline	4-pralines	Calories: **180** | Fat: **15.3g** | Protein: **8.9g** | Total Carbs: **3.2g** | Dietary Fiber: **1.5g** | Net Carbs: **1.7g**	
DINNER	Chickpeas & Carrot Consommé	1-serving bowl	Calories: **460** | Fat: **38.2g** | Protein: **23.3g** | Total Carbs: **10.1g** | Dietary Fiber: **4.3g** | Net Carbs: **5.8g**	
	Cinnamon Cup Cake	1-cup cake	Calories: **263** | Fat: **24.1g** | Protein: **7.6g** | Total Carbs: **14.2g** | Dietary Fiber: **10.3g** | Net Carbs: **3.9g**	
TOTAL CALORIE CONSUMPTION			2,000	
FAT			168.2g	75.7%
PROTEIN			89.4g	17.8%
NET CARBOHYDRATES			32.3g	6.5%

DAY-3	KETOGENIC MEALS	SERVING PORTION	NUTRITIONAL VALUES PER SERVING
BREAKFAST	Ave Avocado Super Smoothie	1-serving bowl	Calories: 398 | Fat: 33.1g | Protein: 20g | Total Carbs: 15.5g | Dietary Fiber: 10.6g | Net Carbs: 4.9g
SNACKS	Tasty Turkey Cheese Cylinders	2-rollups	Calories: 162 | Fat: 10.9g | Protein: 15.6g | Total Carbs: 3.8g | Dietary Fiber: 0g | Net Carbs: 3.8g
LUNCH	Shrimps & Spinach Spaghetti	1-serving plate	Calories: 425 | Fat: 33g | Protein: 25g | Total Carbs: 15.7g | Dietary Fiber: 10.4g | Net Carbs: 5.3g
LUNCH	Chilled Cream	2-ice cream scoops	Calories: 340 | Fat: 34.8g | Protein: 3.7g | Total Carbs: 5.2g | Dietary Fiber: 2.1g | Net Carbs: 3.1g
SNACKS	Philadelphia Potato Praline	4-pralines	Calories: 180 | Fat: 15.3g | Protein: 8.9g | Total Carbs: 3.2g | Dietary Fiber: 1.5g | Net Carbs: 1.7g
DINNER	Charred Chicken with Squash Seed Sauce	2-chicken skewers	Calories: 428 | Fat: 35.6g | Protein: 21g | Total Carbs: 16.9g | Dietary Fiber: 11.6g | Net Carbs: 5.3g
DINNER	Choco 'Cado Twin Truffles	3-candy balls	Calories: 68 | Fat: 5.8g | Protein: 1.6g | Total Carbs: 4.2g | Dietary Fiber: 1.8g | Net Carbs: 2.4g
TOTAL CALORIE CONSUMPTION			2,001
FAT			168.5g — 75.7%
PROTEIN			95.8g — 19.1%
NET CARBOHYDRATES			26.5g — 5.2%

DAY-4	KETOGENIC MEALS	SERVING PORTION	NUTRITIONAL VALUES PER SERVING
BREAKFAST	Coco Cinnamon-Packed Pancakes	2-pancakes	Calories: **392** | Fat: **32.5g** | Protein: **20g** | Total Carbs: **11.3g** | Dietary Fiber: **6.4g** | Net Carbs: **4.9g**
SNACKS	Kingly Kale Crispy Chips	1-serving bowl	Calories: **81** | Fat: **7.6g** | Protein: **1.9g** | Total Carbs: **2.1g** | Dietary Fiber: **0.9g** | Net Carbs: **1.2g**
LUNCH	Bun-less Bacon Burger	1-bacon burger	Calories: **435** | Fat: **36.3g** | Protein: **21.7g** | Total Carbs: **6.1g** | Dietary Fiber: **0.7g** | Net Carbs: **5.4g**
LUNCH	Chocolate-Coated Sweet Strawberries	2-candy cubes	Calories: **125** | Fat: **11.1g** | Protein: **2.7g** | Total Carbs: **5g** | Dietary Fiber: **1.4g** | Net Carbs: **3.6g**
SNACKS	Coconut Candy	4-candy balls	Calories: **204** | Fat: **17.2g** | Protein: **10.2g** | Total Carbs: **3g** | Dietary Fiber: **0.8g** | Net Carbs: **2.2g**
DINNER	Shirataki & Soy Sprouts Pad Thai with Peanut Tidbits	1-serving bowl	Calories: **423** | Fat: **35.2g** | Protein: **21g** | Total Carbs: **14.9g** | Dietary Fiber: **9.6g** | Net Carbs: **5.3g**
DINNER	Chilled Cream	2-ice cream scoops	Calories: **340** | Fat: **34.8g** | Protein: **3.7g** | Total Carbs: **5.2g** | Dietary Fiber: **2.1g** | Net Carbs: **3.1g**
TOTAL CALORIE CONSUMPTION			2,000
FAT			174.7g	78.6%
PROTEIN			81.2g	16.3%
NET CARBOHYDRATES			25.7g	5.1%

DAY-5	KETOGENIC MEALS	SERVING PORTION	NUTRITIONAL VALUES PER SERVING	
BREAKFAST	Chocolate Chia Plain Pudding	1-serving bowl	Calories: 370 | Fat: 28.7g | Protein: 22.3g | Total Carbs: 10.8g | Dietary Fiber: 5.2g | Net Carbs: 5.6g	
SNACKS	Choco Coco Cups	2-mini cups	Calories: 240 | Fat: 25.3g | Protein: 2.1g | Total Carbs: 5g | Dietary Fiber: 4g | Net Carbs: 1g	
LUNCH	Poultry Pâté & Creamy Crackers	3-crackers topped with pate	Calories: 437 | Fat: 36.4g | Protein: 21.9g | Total Carbs: 5.5g | Dietary Fiber: 0g | Net Carbs: 5.5g	
LUNCH	Choco 'Cado Twin Truffles	3-candy balls	Calories: 68 | Fat: 5.8g | Protein: 1.6g | Total Carbs: 4.2g | Dietary Fiber: 1.8g | Net Carbs: 2.4g	
SNACKS	Power-Packed Butter Balls	2-balls	Calories: 128 | Fat: 10.1g | Protein: 4.9g | Total Carbs: 7.2g | Dietary Fiber: 2.9g | Net Carbs: 4.3g	
DINNER	Fresh Fettuccine with Pumpkin Pesto	1-serving bowl	Calories: 417 | Fat: 34.7g | Protein: 20.9g | Total Carbs: 10.5g | Dietary Fiber: 5.3g | Net Carbs: 5.2g	
DINNER	Chilled Cream	2-ice cream scoops	Calories: 340 | Fat: 34.8g | Protein: 3.7g | Total Carbs: 5.2g | Dietary Fiber: 2.1g | Net Carbs: 3.1g	
TOTAL CALORIE CONSUMPTION			2,000	
FAT			175.8g	79.1%
PROTEIN			77.4g	15.5%
NET CARBOHYDRATES			27.1g	5.4%

DAY-6	KETOGENIC MEALS	SERVING PORTION	NUTRITIONAL VALUES PER SERVING
BREAKFAST	Veggie Variety with Peanut Paste	1-serving bowl	Calories: 349 | Fat: 28.7g | Protein: 18.4g | Total Carbs: 10.8g | Dietary Fiber: 6.5g | Net Carbs: 4.3g
SNACKS	Ambrosial Avocado Puree Pudding	1-glass	Calories: 240 | Fat: 23.8g | Protein: 2.8g | Total Carbs: 12.8g | Dietary Fiber: 9g | Net Carbs: 3.8g
LUNCH	Single Skillet Seafood-Filled Frittata	1-frittata wedge	Calories: 459 | Fat: 38.2g | Protein: 22.9g | Total Carbs: 8.7g | Dietary Fiber: 3g | Net Carbs: 5.7g
LUNCH	Carrot Compact Cake	2-cake balls	Calories: 94 | Fat: 8.3g | Protein: 2.8g | Total Carbs: 5.2g | Dietary Fiber: 3.1g | Net Carbs: 2.1g
SNACKS	Philadelphia Potato Praline	4-pralines	Calories: 180 | Fat: 15.3g | Protein: 8.9g | Total Carbs: 3.2g | Dietary Fiber: 1.5g | Net Carbs: 1.7g
DINNER	Therapeutic Turmeric & Shirataki Soup	1-serving bowl	Calories: 415 | Fat: 34.6g | Protein: 21.6g | Total Carbs: 10.1g | Dietary Fiber: 5.7g | Net Carbs: 4.4g
DINNER	Cinnamon Cup Cake	1-cup cake	Calories: 263 | Fat: 24.1g | Protein: 7.6g | Total Carbs: 14.2g | Dietary Fiber: 10.3g | Net Carbs: 3.9g
TOTAL CALORIE CONSUMPTION			2,000
FAT			174.6g — 77.8%
PROTEIN			85.0 g — 17.0%
NET CARBOHYDRATES			25.1g — 5.2%

DAY-7	KETOGENIC MEALS	SERVING PORTION	NUTRITIONAL VALUES PER SERVING	
BREAKFAST	Cream Cheese Protein Pancake	2-pancakes	Calories: **340** | Fat: **28.1g** | Protein: **16.2g** | Total Carbs: **8.1g** | Dietary Fiber: **3.8g** | Net Carbs: **4.3g**	
SNACKS	Power-Packed Butter Balls	2-butter balls	Calories: **128** | Fat: **10.1g** | Protein: **4.9g** | Total Carbs: **7.2g** | Dietary Fiber: **2.9g** | Net Carbs: **4.3g**	
LUNCH	Baked Broccoli in Olive Oil	1-serving bowl	Calories: **484** | Fat: **39.2g** | Protein: **26.7g** | Total Carbs: **21.6g** | Dietary Fiber: **16.8g** | Net Carbs: **4.8g**	
	Cool Cucumber Sushi with Sriracha Sauce	3-sushi slices	Calories: **110** | Fat: **10.1g** | Protein: **1.9g** | Total Carbs: **4.8g** | Dietary Fiber: **2g** | Net Carbs: **2.8g**	
SNACKS	Corndog Clumps	2-corndogs	Calories: **148** | Fat: **13.2g** | Protein: **3.9g** | Total Carbs: **4g** | Dietary Fiber: **1.6g** | Net Carbs: **3.4g**	
DINNER	Roasted Rib-eye Skillet Steak	1-slice rib-eye steak	Calories: **722** | Fat: **60.2g** | Protein: **45g** | Total Carbs: **0g** | Dietary Fiber: **0g** | Net Carbs: **0g**	
	Choco 'Cado Twin Truffles	3-candy balls	Calories: **68** | Fat: **5.8g** | Protein: **1.6g** | Total Carbs: **4.2g** | Dietary Fiber: **1.8g** | Net Carbs: **2.4g**	
TOTAL CALORIE CONSUMPTION			2,000	
FAT			166.7g	75.0%
PROTEIN			100.2 g	20.0%
NET CARBOHYDRATES			22.0g	5.0%

Conclusion

The ketogenic diet is neither a current fad nor a passing trend. Fact is that the ketogenic diet is a lot more powerful than those fundamentals suggested by some trendy and more popular regimen. At present, medical studies and research continue to explore and discover more about nutritional ketosis in particular and the ketogenic diet in general for further benefits and applications that they may bestow to the rest of humankind.

Contrary to what most people and pseudo-experts perceive about the diet, it is also noteworthy that the ketogenic diet is not a high-protein regimen. It is essentially a high-fat diet with a substantially reduced carbohydrate allowance and moderated protein consumptions.

As a summary, the quintessential ketogenic food composition generally consists of smaller quantities of protein, greater contents of organic or natural fats, and ample amounts of dark, green, leafy vegetables. Its concept and working principle behind is to use ketones as an alternative energy source of the body.

Upon digesting foods that contain carbohydrates, your body breaks them down into glucose. With greater carbohydrate consumptions, your blood sugar level increases, indicating an overabundance of glucose. For diabetics, they clearly understand that having high blood sugar levels from eating more carbohydrates is harmful to the body.

Therefore, your intake of more fats and lesser carbohydrates with regulated protein consumptions will eventually result in switching your body's usual metabolism process. In particular, it taps and uses your stored fats to convert them into energy instead of burning glucose or sugar, or generally, carbohydrates. Such a normal metabolic shift creates more ketone bodies while at the same time, lowering blood sugar levels and insulin production in your liver.

As glucose levels drop and ketone bodies increase in number and dominate along your bloodstream, all of your major body organs like your heart, brain, muscles, and other body cells ultimately cease to burn sugar. Left with no choice, they would rather use the ketone bodies as a substitute fuel source that leads to establishing nutritional or optimal ketosis. In other words, your body virtually becomes a fat-burning machine!

Once your body applies the ketones as principal fuel sources, a myriad of beneficial effects ensue. Thus, the bottom line of the ketogenic diet is for you to reap all the rewards of the regimen by simply switching your body to ketosis through altering the way you eat.

When implementing the dietary program properly, the keto diet is capable of being a potent regulator of metabolic disorders. Both anti-oxidant and anti-inflammatory effects of nutritional ketosis alone have always proved to be potent.

Foremost, engaging with the ketone producing, low-carb, and high-fat diet helps to shed off excess weight, strengthen and tone your muscles, enhance your moods, slow down your aging process, lowers your cholesterol levels, and boosting your energy levels.

More importantly, the ketogenic diet creates a massive impact on your general health and wellbeing since it addresses a broad spectrum of health issues, as well as several symptoms associated with inflammatory diseases. Indeed, while you are constantly under the state of ketosis, not only does it augment in the treatment of several serious health problems but also, it enables you to live a more confident, hassle-free, fulfilling and happier life.

To learn how to lose weight and stay fit needs a lot of skill that you will use for a lifetime to keep your body in tip-top shape for the sake of your health and well-being. This book points you towards going to the right direction with a no-arbitrary approach to losing weight in a healthy way. It further provides you with the proper guidance of implementing the regimen via a strategic meal-planning program while using exclusively keto-diet recipes that will enable losing weight in the most natural and simplest way.

Thanks to the proper guidance from a group of certified weight loss experts that the writer collaborated with all this time. You will lose fat and stay fit for life. Have a good luck! Get started with your ketogenic diet! We know you can do it! It is time to shed off those extra pounds. As with any other meal plans, always consult your physician before taking part in a diet plan.

References

[1]USDA Dietary Reference Intakes for Energy, Carbohydrate, Fiber, Fat, Fatty Acids, Cholesterol, Protein, and Amino Acids (page 275)

[2]Hashimoto Y, Fukuda T, Oyabu C, et al. Impact of low-carbohydrate diet on body composition: a meta-analysis of randomized controlled studies. Obes Rev. 2016;17(6):499-509

[3]Bueno NB, De Melo IS, De Oliveira SL, Da Rocha Ataide T. Very-low-carbohydrate ketogenic diet v. low-fat diet for long-term weight loss: a meta-analysis of randomized controlled trials. Br J Nutr. 2013;110(7):1178-87.

[4]Brehm BJ, Seeley RJ, Daniels SR, D'alessio DA. A randomized trial comparing a very low carbohydrate diet and a calorie-restricted low-fat diet on body weight and cardiovascular risk factors in healthy women. J Clin Endocrinol Metab. 2003;88(4):1617-23.

[5]Stern L, Iqbal N, Seshadri P, et al. The effects of low-carbohydrate versus conventional weight loss diets in severely obese adults: one-year follow-up of a randomized trial. Ann Intern Med. 2004;140(10):778-85.

[6]Volek J, Sharman M, Gómez A, et al. Comparison of energy-restricted very low-carbohydrate and low-fat diets on weight loss and body composition in overweight men and women. Nutr Metab (Lond). 2004;1(1):13.

[7]Paoli, A., Bosco, G., Camporesi, E. M., & Mangar, D. (2015). Ketosis, ketogenic diet and food intake control: a complex relationship. Frontiers in psychology, 6, 27.

[8]Paoli, A., Rubini, A., Volek, J. S., & Grimaldi, K. A. (2013). Beyond weight loss: a review of the therapeutic uses of very-low-carbohydrate (ketogenic) diets. European journal of clinical nutrition, 67(8), 789.

[9]Sackner-Bernstein J, Kanter D, Kaul S (2015) Dietary Intervention for Overweight and Obese Adults: Comparison of Low-Carbohydrate and Low-Fat Diets. A Meta-Analysis. PLoS ONE 10(10): e0139817. https://doi.org/10.1371/journal.pone.0139817

[10]Gibson, A. A., Seimon, R. V., Lee, C. M., Ayre, J., Franklin, J., Markovic, T. P., & Sainsbury, A. (2015). Do ketogenic diets really suppress appetite? A systematic review and meta-analysis in obesity reviews, 16(1), 64-76.

[11]Diabetes & Metabolic Syndrome: Clinical Research & Reviews

[12]Feinman RD, Pogozelski WK, Astrup A, et al. Dietary carbohydrate restriction as the first approach in diabetes management: a critical review and evidence base. Nutrition. 2015;31(1):1-13.

[13]Veech, R. L. (2004). The therapeutic implications of ketone bodies: the effects of ketone bodies in pathological conditions: ketosis, ketogenic diet, redox states, insulin resistance, and mitochondrial metabolism, prostaglandins, leukotrienes, and essential fatty acids, 70(3), 309-319.

[14]Hall, K. D., & Guo, J. (2017). Obesity energetics: body weight regulation and the effects of diet composition. Gastroenterology, 152(7), 1718-1727.

[15]Archives of Internal Medicine. 2009 Nov 9; 169(20):1873-80. doi: 10.1001/archinternmed.2009.329. Long-term effects of a very low-carbohydrate diet and a low-fat diet on mood and cognitive function.

Disclaimer

The information contained in **"THE KETO LIFESTYLE"** and its components, means to serve as a comprehensive collection of strategies that the author of this eBook has done research about. Summaries, strategies, tips, and tricks are only recommendations by the author. Reading this eBook will not guarantee that one's results will exactly mirror the author's results.

The author of this eBook has made all reasonable efforts to provide current and accurate information for the readers. The author and its associates shall never be responsible for any unintentional errors or omissions found herein.

The material in the eBook may include information from third parties. Third party materials comprise of opinions expressed by their owners. As such, the author of this eBook does not assume responsibility or liability for any third party material or opinions.

The publication of third party material does not constitute the author's guarantee of any information, products, services, or opinions contained within third party materials. Use of third party materials does not guarantee that your results will mirror our results. Publication of such third party material is simply a recommendation and expression of the author's own opinions of that material.

Whether because of the progression of the Internet or the unforeseen changes in company policies and editorial submission guidelines, stated as fact as of this writing may become outdated or inapplicable later.

This eBook is copyright ©2018 by **Mary Parrett** with all rights reserved. It is illegal to distribute, copy, or create derivative works from this eBook, either in whole or in parts. No parts of this document may be reproduced or retransmitted in any forms whatsoever without the written, expressed, and signed permission from the author.

www.ingramcontent.com/pod-product-compliance
Lightning Source LLC
Chambersburg PA
CBHW061802250726
48657CB00001B/252